GLAUCOMA SURGERY

GLAUCOMA SURGERY

Maurice H. Luntz, M.D.

Professor of Ophthalmology
Mt Sinai School of Medicine
Director of Ophthalmology
Beth Israel Medical Center

Consultant
Manhattan Eye, Ear, & Throat Hospital
New York, New York

Raymond Harrison, M.D.

Attending Surgeon and Director
Glaucoma Service
Manhattan Eye, Ear, & Throat Hospital
New York, New York

Howard I. Schenker, M.D.

Assistant Clinical Professor
University of Rochester
Rochester, New York

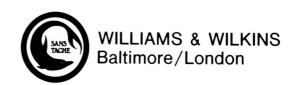

WILLIAMS & WILKINS
Baltimore/London

Editor: Barbara Tansill
Associate Editor: Carol-Lynn Brown
Copy Editor: Deborah K. Tourtlotte
Design: Bert Smith
Illustration Planning: Reginald R. Stanley
Production: Raymond E. Reter

Copyright ©, 1984
Williams & Wilkins
428 East Preston Street
Baltimore, MD 21202, U.S.A.

Accurate indications, adverse reactions, and dosage schedules for drugs are provided
in this book, but it is possible that they may change. The reader is urged to review
the package information data of the manufacturers of the medications mentioned.

Made in the United States of America

Library of Congress Cataloging in Publication Data

Luntz, Maurice
  Glaucoma surgery.

  Bibliography: p.
  includes index.
  1. Glaucoma—Surgery—Atlases. I. Harrison, Raymond.
II. Schenker, Howard. III. Title. [DNLM: 1. Glaucoma—Surgery—Atlases. WW 17
L964a]
RE871.L84 1984   617.7′41059′0222   83-10596
ISBN 0-683-05245-4

Composed and printed at the
Waverly Press, Inc.
Mt. Royal and Guilford Aves.
Baltimore, MD 21202, U.S.A.

to
June, Melvyn, Caryn and David

to
Wilma and David

for
Arlene, Andrew and Emily

Preface

Surgery for congenital and for adult onset glaucomas has advanced considerably since the widespread use of surgical (operating) microscopes. New, effective and safer techniques have resulted in the earlier use of surgery in the treatment of open angle glaucoma. The result of all this has been the need for a restatement of the role of surgery in the treatment of glaucoma, a guide toward selecting the best surgical procedure from those available depending on the clinical circumstances and a detailed description of the most effective surgical techniques.

We have attempted to achieve these goals using an atlas approach. This atlas is not intended to be a comprehensive statement of present-day surgery for glaucoma but rather a guide to the use of surgery in glaucoma with clear and detailed description and illustrations of those surgical procedures we find most effective in differing clinical situations. This should be of value to all ophthalmologists.

The section on congenital, infantile and juvenile glaucoma covers historical perspectives, pathogenesis and clinical entities in greater depth than does the section on adult onset glaucoma. This is deliberate, as it was believed that there is such a paucity of available literature in these areas that they should be dealt with more extensively. However, in keeping with the rest of this atlas, we have emphasized our own concepts and approach to treatment, based on our experience and research.

It is hoped that this atlas will make a positive contribution to the surgical treatment of glaucoma patients.

Acknowledgments

We wish to thank Mrs. Irene Trilling for her secretarial assistance; Mr. Bruce Bailey and Mr. Moses Furman for the photography; Ms. Meryl Greene for the line drawings; and Drs. Howard Jacobson and Jack Greenberg who assisted with the proofreading. We are indebted to our colleagues who shared their patients and to our residents for their thought-provoking questions which made us aware of the need for *Glaucoma Surgery*. We appreciate the valuable assistance of Ms. Barbara Tansill and the staff at Williams & Wilkins during the preparation of this book.

Contents

Section 1   Congenital, Infantile and Juvenile Glaucoma

Section 2   Adult Onset Glaucomas

Section 1

CONGENITAL, INFANTILE AND JUVENILE GLAUCOMA

Maurice H. Luntz, M.D.

Professor of Ophthalmology
Mt. Sinai School of Medicine
Director of Ophthalmology
Beth Israel Medical Center

Consultant
Manhattan Eye, Ear & Throat Hospital
New York, New York

and

Howard I. Schenker, M.D.

Assistant Clinical Professor
University of Rochester
Rochester, New York

Chapter 1

EMERGENCE OF A DISEASE ENTITY

Congenital glaucoma results from a developmental abnormality of the anterior chamber angle. It is an extremely uncommon condition, occurring in about 1:10,000 live births, but it may have significant effects on vision. The outstanding clinical feature is enlargement of the globe which can occur due to distention of the ocular coats by raised intraocular pressure.

The early writers, such as Hippocrates, Celsus and Galen, recognized congenital enlargement of the globe. They did not associate it with elevated intraocular pressure and they included in a single clinical entity all those conditions where the globe appeared to be of unusual size, exophthalmos amongst them. In the 16th century Ambroise Paré (1517–1590) coined the term "ox-eye" to describe the enlargement of the globe: "Oeil de beuf (Bôus ὄφθαλμος) est une maladie d'oeil quand il est gros et eminent, sortant hors la teste, comme on voit les boefs les avoir." In 1722 Saint-Yves attempted to classify the various forms of ocular enlargement in "De la grosseur demesuree du Globe de l'oeil." He included (1) the naturally large eye, (2) exophthalmos and (3) increase in the size of the eye due to an abundance of aqueous humor.

BUPHTHALMOS RELATED TO ELEVATED INTRAOCULAR PRESSURE

The first reference to elevated intraocular pressure in association with enlargement of the globe is credited to Berger in 1744. Despite this, the term buphthalmos was taken to include a variety of conditions such as high myopia, anterior staphylomata and megalocornea. In 1869 von Muralt established the position of classical buphthalmos within the family of glaucoma. Both he and von Graefe (1869) believed that the corneal enlargement was primary and that the ocular hypertension resulted from damage to the corneal nerves. Other authors felt that the glaucoma was secondary to uveal inflammation (Raab, 1876; Gallenga, 1885; Pfluger, 1884; and others).

ABNORMALITIES OF THE ANTERIOR CHAMBER ANGLE

Abnormalities of the anterior chamber angle were being discovered at about the same time (Scheiss-Gemuseus, 1863, 1884; Horner, 1880; Collins, 1896, 1899). In the early part of the 20th century, the changes in the angle were shown to be primary and the inflammatory changes secondary by Reis (1905) and Seefelder (1905). The distinction between a physiologically large eye or cornea and true glaucomatous enlargement of the eye was firmly established by Kayser (1914), Seefelder (1916) and Kestenbaum (1919), as well as others.

An excellent summary of the existing literature and an exhaustive monograph was written by Anderson in 1939. Anderson suggested the term hydrophthalmos be taken as synonymous with congenital glaucoma and that other more colorful terms, including buphthalmos, be discarded.

TREATMENT OF ELEVATED INTRAOCULAR PRESSURE

A new era was introduced by Otto Barkan (1948) who modified a technique first described by de Vincentiis in 1893 and named it "goniotomy." The goniotomy procedure proved to be the first effective method for controlling the intraocular pressure, and it resulted in a significant improvement in the prognosis. In 1960, Redmond Smith introduced the procedure of trabeculotomy ab externo, which brought microsurgical techniques to the treatment of the disease.

BUPHTHALMOS RELATED TO ABNORMALITIES OF THE ANTERIOR CHAMBER ANGLE

The association of abnormalities of the anterior chamber angle and elevated intraocular pressure was made in the late 19th century. These are regarded as developmental anomalies of the angle, present at birth. The disease may manifest at birth, during infancy, or later, or it may remain subclinical depending on the extent of the developmental anomalies.

CONGENITAL, INFANTILE AND JUVENILE GLAUCOMA

"Congenital" glaucoma includes all those patients in whom the clinical features of the disease are present at birth or within 3 months after birth.

Distinction has often been made between those patients presenting before age 3 years and those presenting later. The early cases generally have enlargement of the globe and are designated as "infantile" glaucoma. The later cases do not exhibit enlargement of the globe and are known as "juvenile" glaucoma. Kluyskens (1950) and others have pointed out that the same developmental angle anomalies are responsible for the three types of glaucoma and that a spectrum of disease exists dependent in part on the completeness and degree of the anomaly, irrespective of the age at which the disease process is manifest. The relationship between the appearance of the angle and the prognosis for surgery has been pointed out by Luntz and Livingston (1977) and Luntz (1979a).

CHANGES IN OPTIC NERVE HEAD

The importance of early change in the optic nerve was stressed by Richardson and Shaffer (1966), Shaffer and Heatherington (1969) and others. Earlier authors felt that anterior scleral distention protected the optic nerve from the effects of raised intraocular pressure. Excellent reviews of these conditions have been published by Walton (1979), Kwitko and others.

This section is intended to clarify and define congenital, infantile and juvenile (C.I.J.) glaucoma for the student and practitioner. It will deal with clinical manifestations of the disease, including the various subtypes which come under the heading of C.I.J. glaucoma. Practical aspects of diagnosis and management will be emphasized, and, in particular, great emphasis will be placed on surgical techniques. A brief literature review and historical perspective will be included.

Chapter 2

CONGENITAL, INFANTILE AND JUVENILE (C.I.J.) GLAUCOMA

C.I.J. glaucoma is a term which may be taken to include several entities. We intend it to mean glaucoma which is related to a developmental abnormality in the anterior chamber angle. It is a disease of children and young adults. When it presents in the first 3 months of life or between the first 3 months and 3 years of life, there are often associated anatomic changes in the globe. The former is best considered congenital glaucoma and the latter infantile glaucoma. When the presentation is after 3 years, there are generally no associated changes in the size of the globe. This is considered juvenile glaucoma. There is probably a continuum between infantile and juvenile glaucoma, which may depend on the degree of anomalous development of the angle. The upper age limit for onset of juvenile glaucoma is generally taken to be 35 years. When the onset of glaucoma occurs after this age, it is not usually related to a developmental angle anomaly but is acquired adult onset glaucoma. Juvenile glaucoma of late onset may fall into either of these two types (developmental angle anomaly or acquired disease of the angle), and clinical differentiation depends on gonioscopy. The late onset juvenile glaucoma patient tends to have an angle which resembles that in typical congenital glaucoma. The angle structures, however, tend to continue to develop after birth so that developmental abnormalities in patients with rather late onset juvenile glaucoma may not be as striking. This may add to the difficulty in separating patients with early onset adult open angle glaucoma and late onset juvenile glaucoma based on developmental angle anomalies.

The relationship between juvenile glaucoma of the C.I.J. type and infantile glaucoma is further suggested by many studies of pedigrees which demonstrate cases of both infantile buphthalmos (with enlarged globe) and juvenile glaucoma.

SECONDARY GLAUCOMAS

C.I.J. glaucoma is a primary condition. Glaucoma in the child may also be secondary to other intra- or extraocular conditions. This glaucoma group may simulate primary congenital glaucoma clinically but should be considered distinct. Potential causes of secondary glaucoma in children include retrolental fibroplasia, tumors, inflammation, trauma and medications. There is also a group of patients in whom glaucoma arises from developmental abnormalities of the angle which are part of more generalized problems in development. The angle anomaly in some of these patients is often indistinguishable from that seen in primary congenital glaucoma. Since the glaucoma in these patients arises from angle anomalies, it seems reasonable to consider it primary rather than secondary. On the other hand, it seems prudent to classify these conditions as a separate group because of the extent of other associated developmental abnormalities. Furthermore, some of these patients have angle anomalies which are quite different from those in primary congenital glaucoma.

Included in this group are Marfan's syndrome, homocystinuria, Sturge-Weber disease, von Recklinghausen's disease, aniridia, Lowe's syndrome and the mesodermal dysgeneses, including Axenfeld's syndrome and Rieger's syndrome.

INCIDENCE

Seefelder (1916) found only 46 examples among 129,520 patients in his clinic from 1891 to 1905, a percentage of 0.035. In the Tubingen clinic from

1875 to 1903, the incidence of the disease was 0.079% according to Anderson (1939). Gros found 8 of 12,000 (0.066%) with the disease in a Paris study. Kaminsky (1913) and Janesch (1927) found the disease among 0.041% and 0.032%, respectively, in Breslau patients. In America, Carvill (1932) found an incidence of 0.01% of some 31,648 patients with eye disorders, and Lehrfeld and Reber (1937) similarly found 0.011% among almost a quarter of a million patients. More recent figures do not seem to differ significantly. Walton (1979) reports that an ophthalmologist without subspeciality interest might expect to encounter one new case every 5 to 10 years.

Duke-Elder (1969) points out, however, that although congenital glaucoma is relatively rare, it constitutes a significant percentage of the causes of blindness in children, particularly in the literature which predates current, more effective forms of management. The incidence among the inmates of institutions for the blind has been reported as 9 of 99 by Durr and Schlegtendal (1889) and as 5% by Priestly Smith (1896). Hubner (1926) found an incidence of 2.4% of inmates of German institutes for the blind. Gonin reported a 13.5% incidence in the Lausanne clinic from 1900 to 1925. In 1942 Baillert found a 23% incidence. In America, Lamb (1925) quoted a 5.3% incidence in the Missouri School for the Blind, and Barkan reported almost 7% among blind American children in 1942.

BILATERAL DISEASE

The majority of the cases are bilateral, occurring approximately twice as often as unilateral cases. Anderson (1939) reported an incidence of bilaterality from 60 to 70% among the series of Grosz, Zahn, Seefelder and Janesch (1905). In his own survey, Anderson (1939) found 86% bilaterality. Walton (1979) reports an 80% bilateral occurrence. There may be asymmetrical involvement between the eyes in bilateral cases.

SEX INCIDENCE

There is a striking preference for males in most of the series reported. Anderson quotes a male predominance of from 58.9 to 71% of cases reported by de Grosz (1932), Zahn (1904), Kunzman (1899), Seefelder (1906), Lamb (1925) and Lehrfeld and Reber (1937). A Japanese report suggests this sex incidence may be reversed in that country. More recent reports continue to show a similar male predominance. Kluyskens in 1950 reported 84%, Lister in 1966 reported 70%, and in 1979 Walton reported 65% male incidence.

HEREDITY

The question of heredity is naturally raised by the striking male dominance in most reported series. Most authors have felt that infantile glaucoma is inherited as an autosomal recessive disorder. Anderson agreed with this view after reviewing the literature extant in 1939. Sugar, in the 1950's also believed the disease was recessively inherited.

According to Duke-Elder, the majority of cases are sporadic, but some 12% show a hereditary tendency, generally with autosomal recessive transmission. The trait is regarded as variably penetrant—generally about 40%, according to Westerlund, but in some families it has been reported to be much higher—even 90 or 100%. The incidence of the gene is about 0.028 in the general population. Consanguinity is present as a determining factor in some 8% of pedigrees. As Duke-Elder points out, some cases of direct parent to child transmission may be due to pseudodominance of a recessive trait. On the other hand, he does quote Heath's (1960) report of a family with three successive generations involved, suggesting true dominant inheritance. Jerndal (1972) also reported a family with true dominant inheritance.

Recent reports by Deurenais, Bonaiti et al. (1978) and their colleagues in France suggest that the inheritance of congenital glaucoma may be by more than one mode. Similarly, Merin and Morin (1972) believed that the inheritance of congenital glaucoma was multifactorial, not simply autosomal recessive.

Several studies of identical twins, each having congenital glaucoma, further suggest the hereditary nature of the condition. Patients with congenital glaucoma may respond to topical steroids with an increased intraocular pressure. In contradistinction to adult open angle glaucoma, the parents of patients with infantile glaucoma do not show an increased rate of steroid responsiveness. Although of interest, this does not have any significance regarding inheritance of congenital glaucoma.

AGE OF ONSET

The great majority of cases of congenital glaucoma are probably present within the first month of life. Anderson (1939) collected the combined series of Seefelder (1916) and his own questionnaire series. The age of onset was at birth in 102 patients (40%); it was before 6 months in 86 (34%) and under 1 year in 30 (12%). It was before 6 years of age in 28 (11%) and over 6 years in 5 (2%).

Scheie (1959) reported that the disease was present at birth in 14 of 45 patients and was apparent by age 6 months in 36 of 45 patients. Barkan noted cloudy corneas at birth in 30 of 87 patients. Gros made the diagnosis at birth in 60% of his patients.

The age of onset is somewhat difficult to determine when comparing various reported series because different criteria were used. Many patients presenting to the physicians had symptoms and signs which were initially unrecognized at earlier ages. Nevertheless, the general consensus is that the majority of cases are recognized within the first 6 months of life.

Of patients with juvenile glaucoma, according to Lohlein (1938), 1.3% were recognized before age 5 years. Almost 39% presented between ages 15 and 20, and 21% between ages 20 and 25.

PATHOGENESIS

The etiology of the raised intraocular pressure in congenital glaucoma is the anomalous development of the anterior chamber angle. Anderson (1939), after reviewing the work extant at that time, concluded that "a defect in the meshwork of the angle is the most common cause of interference with the function of the canal of Schlemm." This may be either an absence, undue persistence, or an aberrant growth of the sclero-corneal trabeculae or of the uveal meshwork. Until 1955 the prevailing theory of etiology was that there was abnormally persistent mesodermal tissue present in the angle which interfered with its function. This tissue reduced outflow of aqueous by its presence alone or by its attachment to peripheral iris, resulting in an anterior insertion of the structure. When present as a truly membranous structure, this tissue was known as Barkan's membrane. Surgical cure was believed to result from incision of this tissue, allowing the iris to fall back, thereby giving the aqueous access to the trabecular meshwork.

In 1955 Allen et al. (1955a) proposed a new theory for the development of the anterior chamber angle. It had previously been felt that mesodermal tissue in the angle was normally resorbed, and as a corollary that failure of this process led to the picture seen in congenital glaucoma. They proposed that the angle formed by a simple splitting of two distinct layers of mesodermal tissue. Accordingly, the anterior layer forms the trabecular meshwork while the posterior layer forms the iris and ciliary body. The different adherent properties of the cells and differential growths causes the two regions to separate. They attributed some cases of developmental glaucoma to failure of complete cleavage of the angle structures. This resulted in persistence of tissue which had failed to resorb. They explained the success of goniotomy to surgical completion of the angle cleavage.

In 1959 Maumenee, while agreeing with the cleavage concept of angle development proposed by Allen et al., described a new type of incomplete angle cleavage, resulting in functional defects. He found an anterior insertion of longitudinal and circular bundles of ciliary muscle into trabecular fibers in front of the scleral spur. Because of their abnormal insertion, the contraction of the muscle of the ciliary body results in narrowing of the trabecular spaces.

The pathogenesis of congenital glaucoma is clearly related to diminished outflow facility as a result of abnormal development of the anterior chamber angle. The precise mechanism by which this occurs is uncertain. Whether the abnormal tissue found in the angle is there as a result of faulty cleavage or resorption remains open to question. What role functional defects due to abnormal ciliary body muscle insertion may have is unclear. As suggested by Maumenee, however, this may be an important factor in many cases.

Although Anderson felt that absence of Schlemm's canal is a factor in the pathogenesis of infantile glaucoma, there is little evidence that this is a significant factor in most cases. Both clinically and pathologically, Schlemm's canal is demonstrable except in advanced cases with distorted anatomy and fibrosis.

Chapter 3

CLINICAL MANIFESTATIONS

The diagnosis of infantile glaucoma is usually made easily if one is aware of the characteristic clinical signs and symptoms.

SYMPTOMS

The symptoms of the disease are photophobia, epiphora and blepharospasm.

Photophobia

Photophobia is generally the earliest symptom in a patient in whom the disease is not present at birth. As Scheie points out, mothers often report that this preceded other manifestations of the disease. The photophobia and other symptoms result from the corneal epithelial edema. Initially the photophobia may only be manifest in the presence of bright light, but eventually it may result in the infant being uncomfortable even in a dimly lit room. An effective method of testing for photophobia is to have the parents bring the infant into a room with the lights off. The child is observed as the room lights are switched on. This maneuver is often more effective than trying to shine a bright flashlight into the child's eye. Photophobia is often the first symptom to disappear after the intraocular pressure is controlled. When it persists following surgery, the intraocular pressure has probably not been sufficiently lowered.

Blepharospasm and Epiphora

The blepharospasm and epiphora are also the result of the corneal edema. Although obstruction to the nasolacrimal duct is a more frequent cause of tearing in a young infant, the presence of epiphora and photophobia in a young child must always raise the possibility of congenital glaucoma, regardless of the absence of other objective signs of disease. Further diagnostic work-up is mandatory, including examination under anesthesia.

DIAGNOSTIC WORK-UP

The diagnostic work-up involves a careful evaluation of intraocular pressure, measurement of corneal diameters both longitudinal and horizontal, gonioscopy, retinoscopy and fundus examination. To do this properly in children of 3 years old or less requires examination with a general anesthetic. Between the ages of 3 years and 5 years, a general anesthetic may be necessary depending on the child's cooperation. After 5 years of age, the examination can generally be done without general anesthesia.

The level of intraocular pressure is directly affected by general anesthesia, which generally results in a reading lower than the true pressure. For this reason, each surgeon examining children with this disease has to formulate a standard anesthetic technique so that repeated follow-up measurements can be compared with one another. Preferably, the same anesthetist should be used for every examination. Furthermore, the intraocular pressure readings should be calibrated for the specific anesthetic technique by testing a series of patients who require general anesthesia for any reason and in whom intraocular pressure readings can be taken before and after anesthesia. The absolute lowering of intraocular pressure for the anesthetic technique that has been selected can then be estimated.

We have selected as a standardized anesthetic nitrous oxide and maintenance of anesthesia using halothane without intubation. No other drugs are used during anesthesia. Measurements are taken only when the child has settled into a "steady stage" under anesthesia.

Using this method we regard the upper limit of normal intraocular pressure to be 18 mm Hg using a Schiotz tonometer. Normalization of intraocular pressure is regarded as a recorded Schiotz tonometer pressure of 18 mm Hg or lower, taking an

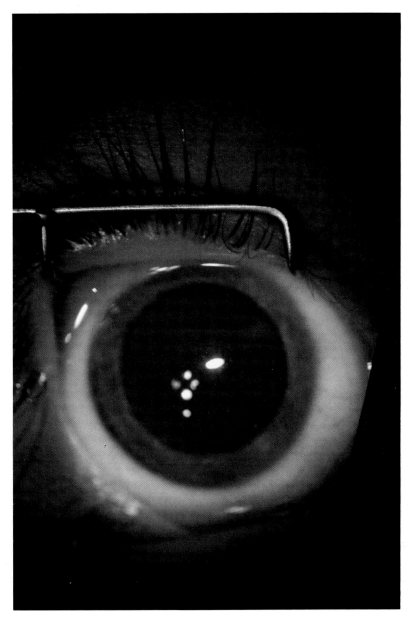

Figure 3.1. C.I.J. glaucoma. A photograph of the eye of a child with C.I.J. glaucoma showing horizontal tears in Descemet's membrane by retro-illumination.

average of scale readings with the 5.5-gm weight and 10-gm weights. The readings should not differ by more than 1 mm Hg.

The Schiotz tonometer is used for the examination under general anesthesia in preference to a hand-held applanation tonometer of which there are a number of choices. In our experience, we have obtained more reproducible and consistent results on repeated examinations at the same sitting and in follow-up measurements with the Schiotz tonometer. Increased corneal diameter does not appear to introduce significant error in the Schiotz measurement.

The other measurements which are made while the child is under general anesthesia are not affected by the anesthesia. The diagnostic work-up should include the evaluation of the following parameters.

Corneal Edema

The most frequent objective sign which brings the patient to the physician is corneal edema. Ini-

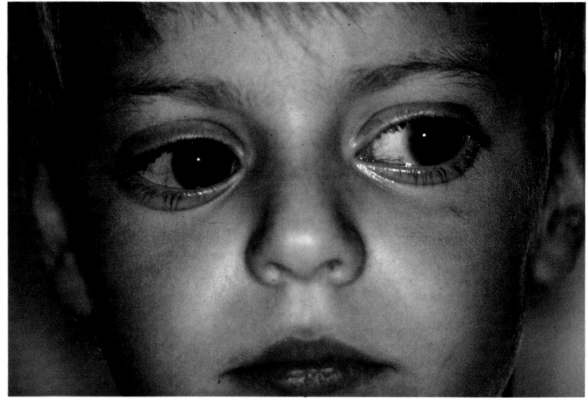

Figure 3.2. C.I.J. glaucoma. Photograph of a young boy with C.I.J. glaucoma showing enlarged corneas in both eyes. There is a good reflex from both corneas, which are not grossly scarred.

tially epithelial, the edema may progress to involve the stroma. Long-standing stromal edema may result in permanent opacities. Corneal clouding may present suddenly, or it may be present at birth in cases where the glaucoma was present in utero. The sudden appearance of corneal edema may represent an acute rise in intraocular pressure. When the edema is epithelial it may come and go as the pressure fluctuates. Sudden decompensation of the corneal endothelium can also cause corneal clouding. The latter may be the result of a break in Descemet's membrane.

Breaks in Descemet's Membrane

These result from the stretching of the cornea in response to the elevated pressure. The breaks tend to be horizontally oriented centrally, and concentric at the limbus; they are usually first found in the lower half of the cornea. They may later involve the upper half of the cornea and may have other orientations than horizontal. They are known as Haab's striae and are best viewed on the slit lamp by retro-illumination (Fig. 3.1).

Enlargement of the Cornea

One of the most striking signs of infantile glaucoma is enlargement of the cornea (buphthalmos)

(Fig. 3.2). It is a direct result of the force of the raised intraocular pressure on the exterior ocular coat. The cornea and sclera are plastic and can stretch until the age of about 3 years.

The normal corneal diameter in infants is between 8 and 10 mm. The horizontal diameter is 0.5 mm longer than the vertical. The period of greatest growth is during the first year of life, at the end of which the diameter may be 11.4 mm. Anderson (1939) quotes a series from Parsons including 20 hydrophthalmic eyes. The smallest horizontal diameter was 12 mm and the largest was 23.5. The average was 16 mm. In nine specimens removed before age 2 ½ years, the average diameter was 12.7 mm; in 31 eyes removed after age 2 ½ years, the average diameter was 15.7 mm. In his own questionnaire series of 110 eyes: 3 were normal, 56 were 12 to 13.75 mm, 43 were 14 to 15.75 and 8 were 16 mm or greater.

The presence of an enlarged cornea (greater than 12 mm) in either the horizontal or the vertical diameter requires further investigation. On the other hand, in the presence of other characteristic signs and symptoms, a normal sized cornea does not exclude the diagnosis. With stretching of the anterior segment, the exact boundaries between cornea and limbus may become indistinct. Contin-

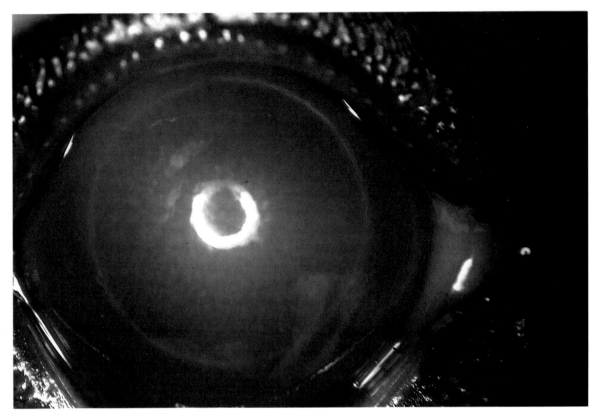

Figure 3.3. C.I.J. glaucoma. A photograph of a buphthalmic eye in a child with C.I.J. glaucoma. The cornea is excessively enlarged and scarred from persistent chronic ocular hypertension.

uing corneal enlargement is a definite sign of congenital glaucoma. Following surgical treatment, further corneal enlargement is a sign of inadequate reduction of pressure.

In addition to an increase in diameter, the cornea undergoes peripheral thinning. According to Anderson, there may be a reversal of the usual relationship between the peripheral and central thickness of the cornea. The cornea also becomes flattened. Gros found an increase from 7.8 to 11.8 mm in corneal radius of curvature. The limbus and adjacent sclera are often thinned as well, and there may be resultant ectasias in this area. In early cases the sclera may actually be thicker than normal posteriorly; the thinning is mainly located anteriorly near the limbus. In the late stages the cornea becomes scarred (Fig. 3.3).

Depth Anterior Chamber

The anterior chamber is characteristically deep. The lens may be as much as 7.3 mm behind the cornea. The entire globe is enlarged in long-standing cases. In a series of 17 eyes, Anderson found an average increase of 5.6 mm in antero-posterior (A-P) diameter, 3.2 mm in horizontal diameter and 2.5 mm in vertical diameter. Globes as large as 44 mm have been reported.

Changes in Refraction

The enlargement of the globe leads to an alteration of the refractive state. The majority of patients are myopic, generally from one to seven diopters. Progressive myopia is an indication that the intraocular pressure is elevated, and the refractive state should be evaluated on each examination. With the marked increase in the A-P diameter of the globe one might expect a greater degree of myopia, but other anatomic factors tend to counteract this. The corneal curvature becomes flatter. In addition the lens become flattened due to stretching of the ciliary body with resulting increased tension on the zonules. Finally, with enlargement of the anterior segment of the globe, the lens is pushed posteriorly. Parsons (1920) calculated that because of these factors, the A-P diameter could increase to 31 mm and the eye still be emmetropic.

Intraocular Pressure

The intraocular pressure must be measured. The intraocular pressure range for the normal newborn is probably similar to that for normal adults. Studies of premature infants suggest that aqueous secretion is low before age 200 days. This implies that patients with symptoms at birth have had elevated pressures for about 2 months in utero. The intraocular pressure in patients with congenital glaucoma is quite often not markedly elevated, although in some cases it may be over 50 mm Hg. A minimally elevated intraocular pressure in the presence of other signs and symptoms is very significant.

The measurement of intraocular pressure in infants is fraught with several sources of error. There is a substantial diurnal variation in pressure in infantile glaucoma. It is possible to miss the peak of pressure and be given a false sense of security. The pressure is generally measured under anesthesia, and most anesthetic agents modify the intraocular pressure. It is necessary, therefore, to develop a standardized technique for examination which will permit valid comparisons. Our recommendations for such a technique are discussed earlier and in Chapter 5. Finally, the method used to measure intraocular pressure may induce inaccuracies. Schiotz tonometry is most often used. Certain assumptions upon which this method depends may not be valid in a buphthalmic eye. The scleral rigidity of the normal infant eye is probably similar to the adult, but this may not be the case when the globe has thinned and enlarged. It is for these reasons that, as stated above, the intraocular pressure measurement must be taken in the context of associated signs and symptoms.

Optic Nerve Head

The optic nerve head in congenital glaucoma is suscpetible to glaucomatous cupping. Originally, it was thought that the distensibility of the anterior portions of the sclera and the cornea protected the nerve from the effects of raised intraocular pressure in the early stages of the disease. More recently the view has arisen that an increase in the size of the cup may arise relatively early in the course of the disease. In normal newborns, Khodadoust et al. (1968) found that only 10% of some 300 patients had cups as large as 0.25, and only 3% had cups larger than 0.5. There was asymmetry between the two eyes in only 3%. Similarly, Richardson and Shaffer (1966) found less than 1% of 520 normal newborns had asymmetry of the cups between their two eyes. On the other hand, pathologic cupping was considered by Shaffer and Hetherington (1969) to be present in some 68% of infantile glaucoma patients by age 12 months. They felt that the infant optic nerve was more susceptible to damage

than the adult nerve because of the lower systemic blood pressure in the infant and that the damage was due to shunting of blood away from the nerve initially, resulting in loss of glia. They also believed that cupping in the infant eye was reversible, and this has been substantiated by other authors. It has been our experience that cupping is often present early on in patients with infantile glaucoma and that it may be reversed following control of intraocular pressure. The reversibility may be due to the fact that early damage is only in the form of glial loss. On the other hand, some authors believe that cupping results from mechanical backward bowing of a weak lamina cribrosa.

Anterior Chamber Angle

The appearance of the angle in infantile glaucoma is crucial for an evaluation of the possible etiology and prognosis for surgery. Appearance of the angle is not sufficient evidence for a diagnosis, however, and must be considered along with other signs and symptoms. A typical angle anomaly may be absent in some cases of glaucoma, or it may be present as an isolated finding without other evidence of disease.

An understanding of the normal gonioscopic appearance of the angle in the newborn is vital to a meaningful assessment of the abnormal angle. The angle in the newborn is not fully developed. The iris inserts in a horizontal plane. Covering the angle structures may be delicate tissue which Barkan (1942) considered to be an endothelial membrane. He called this a chagrined membrane. He felt it covered the uveal meshwork and extended from Schwalbe's line to the peripheral iris. The uveal meshwork is more abundant than in the adult according to Barkan. Other authors consider that the delicate tissue covering the angle is actually the uveal meshwork. Walton (1979) described it as being a homogeneous, gossamer membrane that reaches from the periphery of the iris to the region of Schwalbe's line. This membrane seems to correspond to the endothelial membrane described by Barkan. During development this tissue, whether it be endothelial or uveal, tends to become more fenestrated and open and less evident gonioscopically. The peripheral iris stroma my be thin, in which case it is possible to see the posterior pigment layer, often in a scalloped form. Radial and circumferential vessels are often evident in the iris or ciliary body. Schlemm's canal is evident as a blood-filled column when pressure is applied with the gonioscope and may be wider in the infant.

The angle in infantile glaucoma differs from the

normal angle in several ways. The angle abnormalities may be asymmetric between the two eyes and may not involve the entire circumference of the angle of the eye. The membranous structure covering the angle tends to be more opaque than in normal eyes, being translucent rather than transparent. Beneath this membrane the ciliary body appears thinner and the scleral spur is less distinct. The "take-off" of the iris root may in some cases occur at a higher level than is usual, appearing to arise from the region of the trabecular meshwork. This appearance may be due to abnormal uveal or mesodermal tissue tenting it anteriorly, and iris stroma may extend up to Schwalbe's line. Schlemm's canal is obscured by the overlying tissue but is generally evident with pressure gonioscopy.

In many cases the full blown picture is not seen, and there may be only aggregates of deeply pigmented tissue lying on the iris root. These may represent mesodermal remnants. On the other hand, there are patients with more marked angle anomalies. This group includes patients with very dense uveal meshwork obscuring the underlying angle structures and those where the iris is attached very anteriorly although still to trabecular meshwork. Walton considers these patients to have "congenital" glaucoma with atypical findings. They tend to do poorly with surgery. Luntz described a group of patients with cicatrization of the angle. They showed golden-brown vascularized tissue terminating in a scalloped border raised above the iris root. Segments of the peripheral iris were pulled anteriorly in between which the iris fell back concavely. The trabecular band was narrowed, and Schlemm's canal was displaced anteriorly. This group also did poorly with surgery.

Finally, there are patients with even greater disturbances of development of the anterior chamber angle. These disturbances include iris adherent to the peripheral cornea, abnormalities of Schwalbe's line and maldevelopment of the iris and anterior chamber angle.

The prognosis for surgery is closely related to the type of angle anomaly, and these are classified and discussed in relation to the prognosis for surgery in Chapter 4.

DIAGNOSIS AND DIFFERENTIAL DIAGNOSIS

A definitive diagnosis of C.I.J. glaucoma is usually straightforward. The child presents with an enlarged cornea, an intraocular pressure above 18 mm Hg (under general anesthesia) and abnormal development of the angle. One can generally obtain a history from the parents of photophobia and epiphora.

In a small minority of cases, however, the clinical findings are not so clear and diagnosis may be difficult. We observe the following rules:

In order to make a definitive diagnosis, any two of the following parameters must be present: raised intraocular pressure (higher than 18 mm Hg under general anesthesia); increased horizontal corneal diameter (larger than 10 mm Hg in infants under the age of 6 months; larger than 11 mm Hg in infants between 6 months to 1 year and larger than 12 mm Hg in infants over 1 year); breaks in Descemet's membrane; pathologic glaucomatous cupping of the optic nerve head, indicating the suspicion of visual field loss; progressive enlargement of the cup observed over a period of months; or typical developmental anomalies of the anterior chamber angle. The presence of any one of these abnormal findings should arouse suspicion and mandates a regular (3 month) follow-up evaluation. The presence of any two of these abnormal findings indicates a positive diagnosis of C.I.J. glaucoma. A careful search should also be made for signs of other congenital developmental anomalies which may indicate that the C.I.J. glaucoma is not primary but secondary. One looks for evidence of Marfan's syndrome, homocystinuria (urine examination), Sturge-Weber syndrome, von Recklinghausen's disease, aniridia, Lowe's syndrome (examination of the urine and x-ray of the bones for evidence of rickets). Secondary buphthalmos (buphthalmos associated with one of the afore-mentioned syndromes) has a different prognosis than primary buphthalmos and generally does not respond as well to surgery or to attempts at visual rehabilitation.

The presence of enlarged cornea in the absence of any other positive findings would suggest that the child has megalocornea rather than C.I.J. glaucoma. These children should be closely watched because enlargement of the cornea may precede other positive manifestations of C.I.J. glaucoma by some months.

The refraction is important because an enlarged cornea may be due to congenital myopia, and this must be differentiated from C.I.J. glaucoma. In congenital myopia, the other parameters will be negative, ultrasound examination will demonstrate an enlarged axial length of the globe and the child will be highly myopic by refraction.

SURGERY AND PROGNOSIS

The prognosis in infantile glaucoma changed dramatically with the introduction of goniotomy by

Otto Barkan in 1942. Prior to this the outlook was poor. Anderson (1939) quoted Seefelder as saying that "I know of no case of operated hydrophthalmia where undiminished sight has been retained till later life." In reviewing the series of operation treatments reported by several authors, Anderson found that one patient in three was blind following surgery. One patient in three had visual acuity less than 6/60, and one in three had acuity better than this. After age 25, no patients had better than 6/36 vision. In the collected series of unoperated patients, only one in four had vision better than 6/60. Two of four were blind by the age of 12. Sixty percent of patients aged 25 to 50 were blind. Barkan (1948) reported successful lowering of intraocular pressure in 152 of 196 patients. Other authors have reported similar results with goniotomy.

The introduction of microsurgical techniques in the form of trabeculotomy led to further improvement in the control of intraocular pressure. McPherson (1973) reported a success rate of 12 of 15 and quoted Harms and Dannheim, who had a 27 of 30 success rate. Luntz (1979a) reported a success rate of 96 of 105. Gregersen and Kessing (1977a) compared results obtained by "macrosurgery"—i.e., goniotomy, trephine and diathermy, to those obtained with trabeculotomy. Macrosurgery controlled intraocular pressure in some 61% of eyes, and microsurgery was successful in 100%. They felt that trabeculotomy was more successful when performed as a per primum procedure than after goniotomy.

There may be other factors affecting the prognosis. The age of onset may be a significant factor. The earlier in life the disease presents, the worse the prognosis. On the other hand, surgery is generally more successful when performed as early as possible. Both of these factors are reflected in many reports on goniotomy. It is generally accepted by goniotomists that the procedure does not do well in patients with significant buphthalmos. Barkan felt that patients with corneal diameters greater than 15 mm were not suitable subjects for goniotomy. Similarly, Robertson (1955) reported 13 of 15 successes in nonbuphthalmic eyes compared to only 3 of 10 successes in buphthalmic eyes.

Although other authors have had the impression that corneal enlargement was a poor prognostic factor in trabeculotomy, this has not been our ex-

perience. In a prospective study of 86 eyes treated by trabeculotomy, the corneal diameter was of no prognostic significance.

Another factor which may be of great prognostic significance is the appearance of the anterior chamber angle. In a study of 86 eyes undergoing trabeculotomy, it was found that eyes with typical angle anomalies did very well. Patients whose angles appeared cicatrized or had evidence of irido-corneal dysgenesis did poorly. The first group had 100% success rate, compared to only about 30% success rates in the latter two groups. These angle anomalies are described in the following chapter.

The successful control of the disease must not be confused with successful control of intraocular pressure. In a review of the long term functional results in patients treated by goniotomy, Richardson et al. (1964) found the following. The intraocular pressure was controlled in 92% of 54 patients. Of these, only 39% had visual acuity of 20/20 to 20/50. Thirty-nine percent had acuity less than 20/200. Of 47 patients with bilateral adequate intraocular pressure control, only 60% had better than 20/50 vision. There was anisometropia and heterotropia in 65%. Damage to the disc was the basis for diminished vision in only 26%.

Corneal scarring, altered refraction, anisometropia and resultant amblyopia all contribute to a poor visual prognosis. The earlier the diagnosis can be made, the better the physician is able to prevent these problems from occurring.

The pathologic findings in congenital glaucoma reflect the changes produced by elevated pressure in the developing eye. There is enlargement and thinning of the cornea and limbus as described above. There is cupping of the optic nerve head with loss of ganglion cells in the retina. Late manifestations include fibrosis of the iris root and trabecular meshwork. The angle demonstrates findings which have been discussed above. These include anterior insertion of the iris, anteriorly displaced ciliary processes, and insertion of the longitudinal displaced ciliary processes, and insertion of the longitudinal and circular ciliary muscles into the trabecular sheet. The canal of Schlemm is present in early cases but may be difficult to demonstrate, particularly in advanced cases, mainly due to collapse of the inner wall onto the outer wall of the canal.

Chapter 4

MANAGEMENT OF C.I.J. GLAUCOMA AND THE PROGNOSIS FOR SURGERY

The prognosis for surgery has already been discussed in general terms in Chapter 3. Following is a discussion of trabeculotomy and, where indicated, trabeculectomy for C.I.J. glucoma and the prognosis related specifically to these surgical techniques. The surgical method will be described in detail.

The management of C.I.J. glaucoma is long term and complex. There are two major aspects to the treatment of the disease: (1) lifetime control of the raised intraocular pressure and (2) visual rehabilitation of the eye once intraocular pressure has been controlled.

Life-long control of the intraocular pressure requires surgery because miotics or mydriatics are not effective as long term methods of treatment, and acetazolamide (Diamox) is generally contraindicated for lifetime use.

The preferred operation is trabeculotomy, which has a number of major advantages over the alternative operation of goniotomy:

1. Trabeculotomy has a documented higher success rate than goniotomy. The latter will control intraocular pressure in about 74% of eyes having glaucoma of all degrees of severity, although there are claims for 85% control if eyes with corneal cloudiness are excluded. Trabeculotomy, on the other hand, will control intraocular pressures in over 90% (McPherson, 1973; Gregersen and Kessing, 1977a; Luntz, 1979a) of eyes with glaucoma of all degrees of severity.

2. Trabeculotomy is technically easier for a well trained microsurgeon because it does not require the introduction of sharp instruments across the anterior chamber, which increases the risk of damage to other ocular tissue. It can be performed with undiminished accuracy in advanced cases where the cornea is edematous or scarred and where there is poor visibility in the anterior chamber.

3. There is no need for the surgeon to adapt to the visual distortion produced by the operating gonioprism.

4. A trabeculotomy is anatomically more precise in creating an opening between the anterior chamber and Schlemm's canal.

5. The success of trabeculotomy depends only on the type of angle anomaly and is not dependent on the severity of the glaucoma, the size of the cornea or the presence of corneal edema—all factors which influence the success of goniotomy.

Trabeculotomy is also the operation of choice rather than goniotomy in those cases which are known to have a good prognosis with trabeculotomy (group 1 angle anomalies as described below). Trabeculotomy produces less surgical trauma and the anterior chamber is entered only briefly. There is a lower incidence of postoperative cataract and a much lower possibility of postoperative complications.

On the other hand, in eyes with a cicatrized angle or frank irido-corneal dysgenesis, trabeculotomy gives such poor results that it is not the procedure of choice. In these eyes, trabeculectomy or combined trabeculotomy with trabeculectomy gives the best long term results. Nevertheless, these results are poor.

Unguarded filtration operations—for example, the Scheie procedure, Elliot's trephine or iridencleisis—have even poorer long term results and should not be used. When a trabeculectomy has failed in eyes with a poor prognosis, then an implanted drainage tube or a cyclocryotherapy is indicated.

Trabeculotomy has a high rate of success in selected eyes (over 90%). The most important determinant for its prognosis is the type of developmental anomaly in the angle (Luntz, 1979a). There follows a description of the angle anomalies seen in C.I.J. glaucoma and their classification based on the ability of trabeculotomy to achieve and maintain normal intraocular pressure.

MESODERMAL ANOMALIES OF THE ANTERIOR CHAMBER ANGLE

The appearance of the anterior chamber angle by gonioscopy shows considerable variation in eyes with glaucoma caused by congenital or developmental anomalies. These angle anomalies fall easily into three major groups, based on the interpretation of the gonioscopic appearance: (1) a major group of angles in which there appears to be a deposit or remnant of mesoderm straddling the trabeculum, ciliary body and root of the iris; (2) a second group that seems to represent the end result of a cicatricial process within the angle and (3) a third group of frank irido-corneal dysgenesis. Furthermore, the results of trabeculotomy, in terms of the control of intraocular pressure, correlate well with this classification. Various angles with a presumed mesodermal anomaly do extremely well with trabeculotomy, whereas the other two groups respond badly.

Group 1: Presumed Mesodermal Anomaly of the Angle

This constitutes the commonest anomaly seen in children with C.I.J. glaucoma, accounting for 73% of the eyes in our series of 105 eyes. This is a large group with three major subdivisions which will be described and illustrated in detail. These differences relate to the consistency, distribution and pigmentation of the mesoderm in the angle. Throughout this group, however, the surface of the iris is flat and normal in appearance. There is no evidence of undulation or of abnormality of the iris surface, which is a characteristic feature of the other two groups. This is a major point of differentiation because it implies that there is no active cicatricial process occurring in the angle, but that the mesodermal anomaly is due to either a deposition of mesoderm or a remnant of mesoderm without any change within the rest of the angle structure. The flatness of the iris surface is recognized by noting that the iris surface is evenly illuminated when the slit lamp beam is focused on it. On careful examination of the iris surface, it is noted to be of

normal structure and consistency, even in its periphery.

SUBGROUP 1

The mesodermal anomaly is manifest as a continuous sheet of mesoderm which stretches from the iris root across the ciliary body, obscures the trabeculum and reaches Schwalbe's line or just beyond. The sheet of mesoderm varies in different eyes in consistency and pigmentation. At one extreme, it is seen as a fine grayish-colored membrane stretching across the angle (Fig. 4.1) and at the

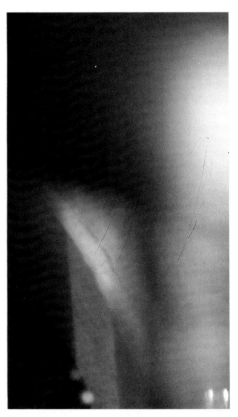

Figure 4.1. Presumed mesodermal anomaly of the angle. Gonioscopic slit lamp view of the anterior chamber angle of a child with C.I.J. glaucoma and a presumed mesodermal anomaly of the angle with minimal pigmentation. In the lower half of the figure the slit lamp beam traverses the iris surface, which is flat and does not undulate. Looking along the iris surface to the center of the photograph, one sees the trabecular band illuminated in the slit lamp beam. The trabecular meshwork is greyish in appearance; the anterior pigmented line is Schwalbe's line.

This type of mesodermal anomaly is infrequently seen in developmental anomalies of the angle and closely resembles the original description of Barkan's membrane. The prognosis for surgery is excellent.

other extreme as a densely pigmented, brown- or black-colored band of mesoderm (Fig. 4.2). This anomaly is seen in 11 of the 86 eyes that we studied.

Figures 4.1 and 4.2 represent gonioscopic views of the angle anomaly. The slit lamp beam illuminates the posterior surface of the cornea where no abnormality is visible. Running one's eye downward from the top of the photograph, the next major structure is the trabecular area, which is seen in Figure 4.1 as a lightly pigmented band of mesoderm and in Figure 4.2 as a densely pigmented, thicker band of tissue. These tissue bands are presumed to be embryonal mesoderm. They extend from Schwalbe's line across the trabecular meshwork, obscuring trabecular landmarks, and on to the iris root. Still looking downward along the slit lamp beam, the next structure, seen particularly in Figure 4.2, is the flat surface of the iris. Note that the iris surface is evenly illuminated by the slit lamp beam and the structure and consistency of the peripheral iris are normal, unchanged from the appearance of the iris closer to the pupil.

SUBGROUP 2

The mesoderm in the angle is fragmented into fine or thick processes, giving a rather different gonioscopic appearance from that seen in subgroup 1. This is seen in Figure 4.3 which illustrates the gonioscopic slit lamp appearance of this anomaly.

At the top of the photograph, the slit lamp beam illuminates the posterior corneal surface, which is normal. Looking down along the posterior corneal surface, the next major structure is a pinkish-colored trabecular band which extends from the root of the iris onto the posterior corneal surface. Crossing the trabecular band are fine processes of mesoderm (iris processes) which appear to rest on the trabecular meshwork. These processes vary in thickness and have a dendritic pattern. Another feature is that the trabecular band is narrow and no ciliary body band is visible, thus indicating that the iris root inserts directly into the base of the trabecular meshwork. This represents an anteriorly placed iris.

In common with the major subgroup, the iris surface is evenly illuminated by the slit lamp beam, indicating that it is flat, and it appears to be normal in structure and consistency.

Seventeen of the 86 eyes studied demonstrated this type of angle anomaly.

SUBGROUP 3

This is another variation of the mesodermal anomaly. In this group, aggregations of deeply pigmented mesoderm lie on the iris root over the ciliary body band and the trabeculum. The anomaly is illustrated in Figure 4.4.

At the top of this figure, the slit lamp beam

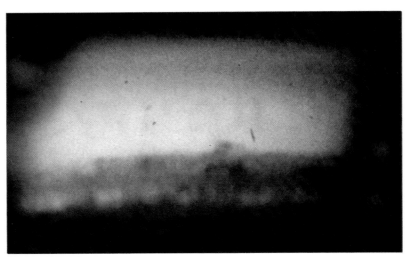

Figure 4.2. Presumed mesodermal anomaly of the angle. Gonioscopic slit lamp view of the anterior chamber angle of a child with C.I.J. glaucoma and a presumed mesodermal anomaly of the angle. At the top of the figure, the slip lamp beam illuminates the posterior surface of the cornea. Below this, the next major structure is the trabecular area seen as a darkly pigmented band of tissue, presumably mesoderm. Looking downward in the slip lamp beam of light, the next structure is the flat surface of the iris, which is evenly illuminated by the light of the slit lamp beam.

The prognosis for the control of intraocular pressure with trabeculotomy in this type of angle anomaly is excellent, with a success rate approaching 100%.

Figure 4.3. Presumed mesodermal anomaly of the angle. The posterior corneal surface is illuminated in the upper portion of the photograph and is normal. The lower half of the slide is a uniform brown color, and this is the surface of the iris. At the junction of the iris and cornea, approximately in the center of the slide, is a pinkish-colored band which is the trabeculum. This extends from the root of the iris onto the posterior corneal surface. Crossing this pinkish trabecular band are fine processes of mesoderm (iris processes) which lie on the trabecular meshwork. These processes vary in thickness and have a dendritic pattern. They all run across the band of trabecular tissue. Another feature is that the trabecular band is rather narrow and no ciliary band is visible. This means that the iris root inserts directly into the base of the meshwork; this represents an anteriorly placed iris. The iris surface is evenly illuminated by the slip lamp beam, indicating that it is flat; therefore, there is no cicatricial process on the iris surface.

The prognosis for control of intraocular pressure with this type of angle anomaly is excellent, with a success rate approaching 100%.

illuminates the posterior surface of the cornea, which appears normal. Looking downward from the posterior corneal surface, the next major structure is the trabeculum area and overlying aggregates of the same darkly pigmented tissue. There is densely pigmented mesoderm lying on the root of the iris, across the trabecular meshwork and extending to Schwalbe's line. Between the aggregates of mesoderm is a band of lighter pigmented mesoderm resting on the trabecular meshwork, and in this area Schwalbe's line is faintly visible. Looking downward from the base of the trabecular meshwork band, one sees the root of the iris. The peripheral iris surface is evenly illuminated by the light of the slit lamp beam and appears normal in structure and contour.

The interpretation of this appearance in the angle is that there is a deposit of darkly pigmented mesoderm resting on the trabecular meshwork and on the root of the iris in the angle. It stretches as a band over the trabecular meshwork, intermittently aggregated into clumps. There is no fibrosis in the iris surface. In the center of the iris surface is a round, brown nodule which is an iris nevus and is an incidental finding.

There were 28 eyes in this subgroup.

SUBGROUP 4

There is a fourth subgroup within this major grouping which constitutes a transitional type. The mesodermal anomaly of the angle is different from the preceding subgroup in the sense that it extends onto the peripheral iris surface, a feature which is not seen in the previous three subgroups but is characteristic of a cicatrized angle, which will be discussed in the next group. This subgroup, however, has in common with the preceding subgroup the observation that the iris surface is flat and appears normal. This is not the case in angles that are cicatrized. The interpretation of this anomaly is that mesoderm has been deposited in the angle or embryonal remnants are present in the angle without any other disease process occurring within the angle. As expected, therefore, the prognosis for surgery in this subgroup is similarly excellent to that in the preceding subgroups and much better than the prognosis in a cicatrized angle.

This type of angle is illustrated in Figure 4.5, which represents the gonioscopic view of the angle. At the top of the illustration, one sees the posterior cornea, which is normal. Looking downward, the next major structure is a band of light brown, almost golden-colored membrane which obscures the trabeculum and can be followed down to the iris root where it has a scalloped border with processes extending onto the peripheral iris surface. These fine processes rest on the peripheral iris surface, but the latter is noted to be flat, evenly illuminated by the slit lamp beam and evidently normal in structure, contour and consistency.

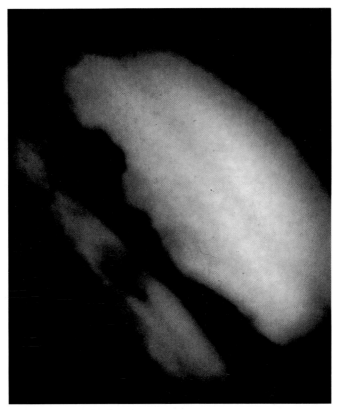

Figure 4.4. Presumed mesodermal anomaly of the angle. No abnormality is visible in the posterior corneal surface (uppermost). The trabecular zone lies approximately in the center of the slit lamp beam. It is characterized by a darkly pigmented band, presumably mesoderm, lying on the trabecular meshwork with scattered aggregates of the same darkly pigmented tissue at each side of the slit lamp beam. This dark mesoderm is lying on the root of the iris and over the trabeculum. Between the two aggregates of the mesoderm on each side of the slit lamp beam is a band of lighter pigmented tissue on the trabecular meshwork, and in this area Schwalbe's line is faintly visible.

Looking down from the base of the trabecular band, one sees the iris surface. The iris surface is evenly illuminated by the light of the slip lamp beam, which indicates that it is flat and no one part of the iris surface is displaced anteriorly or posteriorly compared to the rest. This is an important point to appreciate because it means that there is no cicatricial component on the iris surface.

The interpretation of this appearance in the angle is that there is a deposit of darkly pigmented mesoderm lying on the trabecular meshwork and on the root of the iris in the angle. It stretches as a band over the trabecular tissue intermittently aggregated into clumps. There is no fibrosis on the iris surface, which is flat and does not undulate.

Peripheral iris: In the center of the iris surface is a round brown nodule which is an iris nevus. The prognosis for surgery is excellent, approaching 100% success rate.

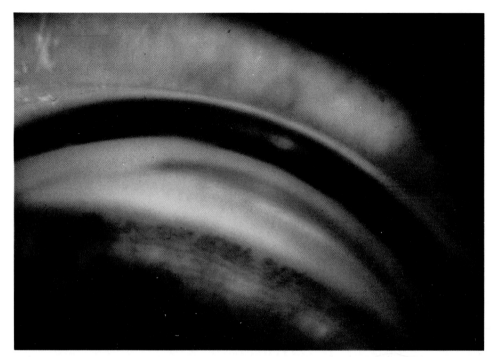

Figure 4.5. Gonioscopic view of a mesodermal anomaly of the angle in a child with C.I.J. glaucoma. This view represents an intermediate stage between a mesodermal anomaly and a cicatrized angle. At the top of the photograph one notes the posterior corneal surface. Looking downward, one sees a brownish membrane across the trabecular zone with stellate processes extending onto the peripheral iris surface. The peripheral iris surface is noted to be evenly illuminated by the slit lamp beam and is not undulating. The prognosis for surgery is similar to that described for other mesodermal anomalies.

There were 17 eyes in this subgroup.

The 73 eyes that constituted this major group of mesodermal anomalies had excellent results with trabeculotomy. These results will be described later in this chapter.

Group 2: Cicatrized Angles

This group of anomalies is characterized by structural changes within the angle, suggesting that a cicatricial process has occurred. The prognosis for surgery in these angles is considerably worse than in those described in the preceding group.

Unlike the previous group, the gonioscopic appearance of the angle in these eyes is relatively uniform, as illustrated in Figure 4.6.

At the top of the illustration, the slit lamp beam illuminates the posterior corneal surface, which is normal. Looking downward, one follows the posterior corneal surface and reaches a dark brown, semicircular band lying within the posterior corneal surface. This is an artifact and should be disregarded. Continuing down, one sees a faint brown line which is Schwalbe's line, the anterior limit of the trabecular meshwork. The trabeculum area below Schwalbe's line is only faintly visible and is remarkable only for the presence of a light brown

membrane at its base. The upper peripheral edge of this membrane is straight and attached to the base of the trabecular meshwork, whereas the lower or free edge has a serrated contour and develops a number of small projections, each of which extends downward onto the surface of the iris root. The apex of some of these projections becomes continuous with a radial fold of iris tissue.

In this manner, the upper half of the iris (that portion of the iris adjacent to the light brown membrane) is divided into a series of radial folds. Thus, the iris, which is at the bottom half of the illustration, can be divided into two parts. The most peripheral part of the iris develops a number of radial folds; between these radial folds, the iris surface forms troughs which lie in a plane posterior to the radial folds. The more central part of the iris is evenly illuminated by the slit lamp beam and is flat.

In the illustration, the peripheral part of the iris is illuminated by the microscope light, which is focused onto the brown membrane at the trabecular meshwork. The light also illuminates the radial folds of the iris so that these folds are in the same horizontal plane as the membrane at the base of the trabecular meshwork. In between these folds of

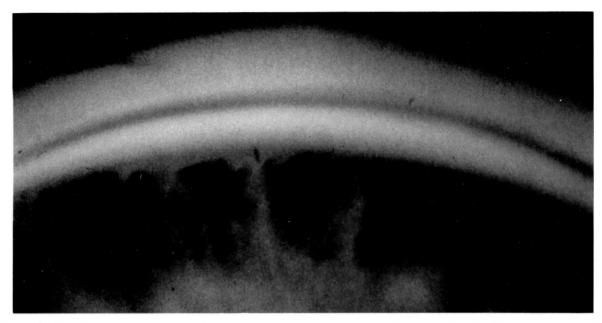

Figure 4.6. Cicatrized angle. Gonioscopic view of a cicatrized angle in a child with C.I.J. glaucoma. The slide should be examined from the top, where the slit lamp beam illuminates the posterior corneal surface. Looking downward, one follows the posterior corneal surface until reaching a dark brown, semicircular band. This is an artifact and should be disregarded. Continuing down, one can see a faint brown line, which is Schwalbe's line, and below it the trabeculum band. Still looking downward, the first prominent structure is a light brown membrane situated on the base of the trabecular meshwork and on the iris root.

The upper or peripheral edge of this membrane is straight and attached to the base of the trabecular meshwork, but the lower or free edge of membrane has a serrated contour and develops a number of small projections, each of which projects downward onto the surface of the iris root. The apex of some of these projections becomes continuous with radial folds of the iris tissue.

These radial folds of iris are illuminated by the microscope light which is focused on the light brown membrane at the trabecular zone. Therefore, these iris folds lie on the same horizontal plane as the membrane attached to the base of the trabecular zone.

In between these folds of iris, the iris surface is dark because it is out of focus and not at the same level as the folds. These darker areas in between the iris folds represent troughs of the iris surface situated at a level posterior to the radial folds that, therefore, are not illuminated by the light of the microscope. If the iris were cut in cross section, the iris surface would undulate the radial folds lying anterior to the rest of the iris surface. The irregular appearance of the iris surface is believed to have resulted from a cicatricial process which affected the angle during its development. The whole limbal area is involved because Schlemm's canal is closer to the limbus in these eyes, situated 0.5 mm to 1.0 mm behind the surgical limbus (conjunctivo-corneal junction) instead of its usual position 2 mm behind the surgical limbus.

Prognosis for trabeculectomy in this type of angle anomaly is poor, with a success rate of about 30%. Trabeculectomy or combined trabeculectomy-trabeculotomy is the surgery of choice.

iris, however, the iris surface is dark and out of focus. These dark areas in between the iris folds are troughs of the iris surface situated at a level posterior to the radial folds, so that if the iris were cut in cross section, the iris surface would be seen to undulate.

The appearance of this angle is interpreted as indicating that the radial folds of iris are situated on the same plane as the light brown membrane which straddles the trabecular meshwork and the iris root. Therefore, the iris surface represented by these radial folds has been pulled to a more anterior level than the iris which lies between these folds. This is presumably the result of a cicatricial process in the angle which is related to the light brown membrane because one can see iris folds connected to the projections of this membrane. In Figure 4.6, on looking from left to right, one can count five to six radial folds of iris that are well illuminated. Similar examples of this angle anomaly, with the same characteristics, are seen in Figures 4.7 and 4.8.

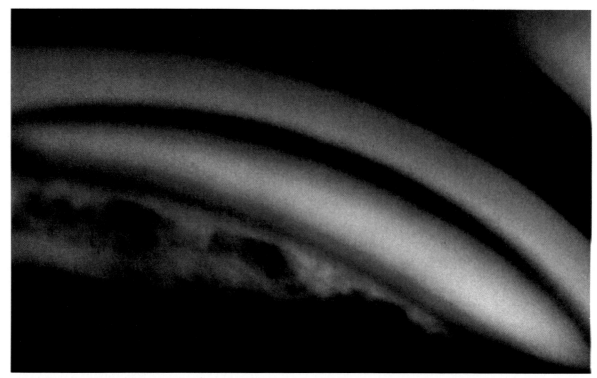

Figure 4.7. Another photograph of a cicatrized angle similar to Figure 4.6. Note the stellate-bordered whitish membrane attached to the trabecular meshwork which sends processes into the peripheral iris surface. The peripheral iris surface undulates as in the previous figure, with troughs of the iris surface in between these processes.

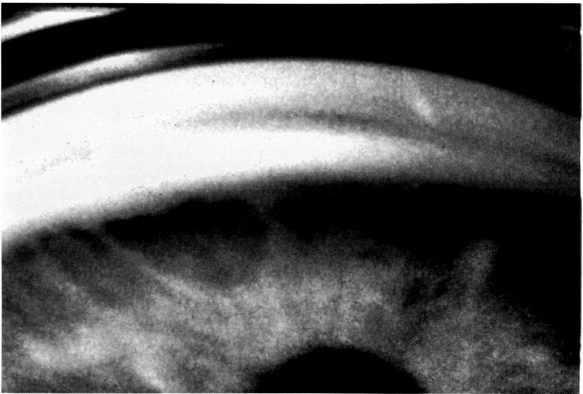

Figure 4.8. Another example of a cicatrized angle seen gonioscopically in a child with C.I.J. glaucoma. In this example, there is a rather narrow brownish membrane attached to the trabecular area with a stellate border along the iris surface and radial folds of iris where the iris is hitched forward by the trabecular membrane. In the center of the picture two radial folds join to form a semicircular iris fold.

Group 3: Irido-corneal Dysgenesis

This group is characterized by varying degrees of angle irido-corneal dysgenesis from mild to severe forms, present in the first few weeks of life. These eyes are characterized by central corneal opacification, prominence of Schwalbe's line—which is anteriorly placed and visible in the cornea due to an abnormally widened trabecular meshwork—and varying degrees of anterior segment malformation. In severe cases, there are adhesions between iris surface at and adjacent to the pupil, the lens capsule or the posterior cornea. A mild form of irido-corneal dysgenesis is seen in Figure 4.9, which demonstrates a prominent Schwalbe's line in the peripheral cornea and obvious structural abnormalities of the iris surface in the periphery. The characteristic angle anomaly is shown in Figure 4.10. At the top of the figure, the slit lamp beam illuminates the posterior corneal surface, which is normal. Looking down, the next major structure is a thickened Schwalbe's line, which is also anteriorly placed in the cornea. Below Schwalbe's line is an abnormally widened trabeculum which looks structureless and in which scattered small pigment deposits are visible. As there is no real structure to the trabeculum, the

sclera is visible through the atrophic trabecular tissue, which looks white. Below the trabeculum is the iris root, which looks flat and is not cicatrized.

A more severe form of the disease is illustrated in Figure 4.11 in which gross structural abnormalities of the cornea and anterior segment of the eye have occurred. Eyes in this group have a poor prognosis for trabeculotomy, rather similar to the eyes in the cicatrized group.

SECONDARY CONGENITAL, INFANTILE AND JUVENILE GLAUCOMAS

These are rare, the commonest examples of which are glaucoma associated with Sturge-Weber syndrome and neurofibromatosis.

Sturge-Weber Syndrome

This is characterized by a port wine stain of the face in the distribution of the fifth cranial nerve (Fig. 4.12). The deformity may involve the angle, causing glaucoma. A mesodermal anomaly similar to that in primary C.I.J. glaucoma is the usual defect (Fig. 4.13). For these patients trabeculotomy is the operation of choice, with good results. In some cases a vascularized membrane forms in the

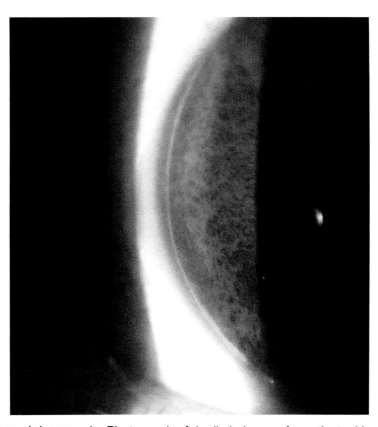

Figure 4.9. Irido-corneal dysgenesis. Photograph of the limbal area of a patient with posterior embryotoxin (a mild form of irido-corneal dysgenesis). The anteriorly placed and thickened Schwalbe's line can be seen near the limbus within the cornea in the slit lamp beam.

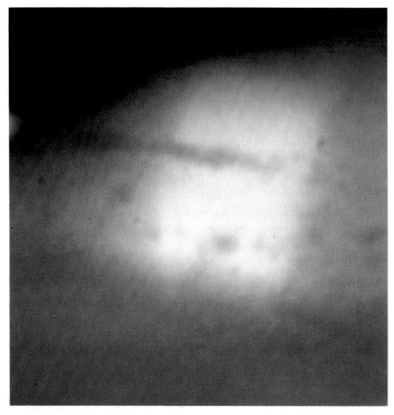

Figure 4.10. Photomicrograph of gonioscopy of a child with advanced irido-corneal dysgenesis with the slit lamp beam illuminating the trabecular area. The trabecular area is noted to be wide, with Schwalbe's line anteriorly placed. Schwalbe's line is recognized as a pigment band in the posterior corneal surface toward the top of the slip lamp beam. The rest of the trabecular area behind Schwalbe's line is pale, with small aggregations of pigment. The entire trabecular meshwork appears to be underdeveloped and featureless. Prognosis for trabeculotomy is poor (30%).

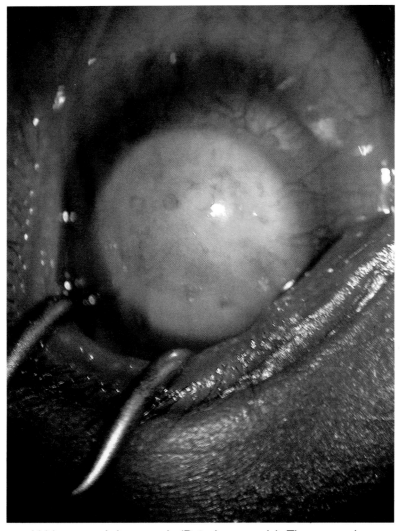

Figure 4.11. Advanced irido-corneal dysgenesis (Peter's anomaly). The cornea is scarred, and the iris and lens are adherent to the posterior corneal surface. Prognosis for trabeculotomy is poor (30%).

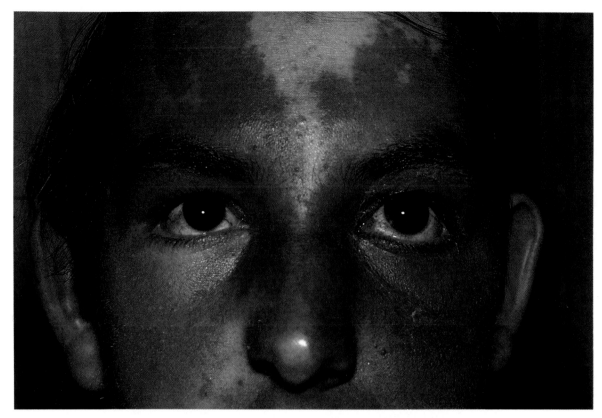

Figure 4.12. Photograph of an adolescent with Sturge-Weber syndrome affecting both sides of his face.

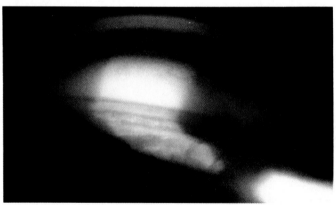

Figure 4.13. Photomicrograph of gonioscopic appearance of the angle in an adolescent with Sturge-Weber syndrome showing a deposit of brownish mesoderm in the trabecular area. The slit lamp beam illuminates the iris surface at the bottom of the photograph, running over the trabecular meshwork in the center of the photograph and then anteriorly onto the posterior corneal surface.

angle (Fig. 4.14). These patients have a poor prognosis for surgery but do better with trabeculectomy than trabeculotomy. If this fails, a seton should be tried (see Chapter 7).

In other cases, the angle appears normal and surgical intervention has uncertain results. The raised intraocular pressure in these eyes could be from raised episcleral venous pressure due to abnormality of the episcleral plexus.

Neurofibromatosis

Neurofibromatosis of the anterior chamber angle has a poor prognosis for surgery. Medical control should be tried initially. When surgery is required, a trabeculectomy is preferable; if that fails, a seton implant may be necessary.

SURGICAL TECHNIQUE WITH TRABECULOTOMY

General anesthesia is used without muscle relaxants. Intubation is generally advisable because the procedure takes at least ½ hour.

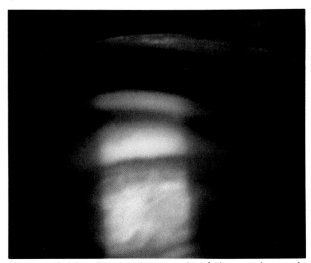

Figure 4.14. Photomicrograph of the gonioscopic appearance of a young child with Sturge-Weber syndrome showing blood vessels in the trabecular area. Looking at the uppermost portion of the slit lamp beam, one is looking at the posterior surface of the cornea. Moving downward, there is a red band which represents the trabecular meshwork suffused with congested blood vessels. Beneath this is the iris surface.

A careful assessment of the intraocular pressure, the corneal diameter, the clinical state of the cornea, the appearance of the iris and lens and the gonioscopic appearance of the angle must be made if this has not already been done. The choice of trabeculotomy as the surgical procedure will depend on the type of angle anomaly present.

The initial cleaning of the eye for surgery and sterile draping is done in the standard fashion, depending on the surgeon's specific routine. Exposure of the eye is achieved by the use of a wire speculum. Neosporin antibiotic drops should be instilled into the conjunctival sac at this point. There is no need for the use of a mydriatic or miotic.

CONJUNCTIVAL FLAP (5× MAGNIFICATION)

The operation is commenced by raising a fornix-based conjunctival flap of 7 mm at the limbus. The dissection is continued to the sclera, raising conjunctiva, Tenon's fascia and episclera. In this manner, a triangular portion of sclera is exposed, measuring at least 3 mm from its base at the surgical limbus to its apex. The surface of the sclera is cleaned.

To rotate the globe, if necessary, 4-0 Mersilene sutures are passed through lamellar thickness of sclera at the edge of the conjunctival flap at the surgical limbus (Fig. 4.15).

SCLERAL DISSECTION (10× MAGNIFICATION)

Using a sharp knife with a microblade, an incision is made through half the scleral depth, extend-

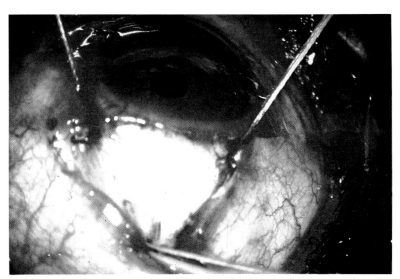

Figure 4.15. Technique for trabeculotomy. A 7-mm wide fornix-based conjunctival flap is raised and dissected as far back as it will go, leaving at least 3 mm of sclera exposed behind the limbus. The eye is stabilized by two 4-0 Mersilene sutures in the episclera at the limbus at each edge of the conjunctival flap.

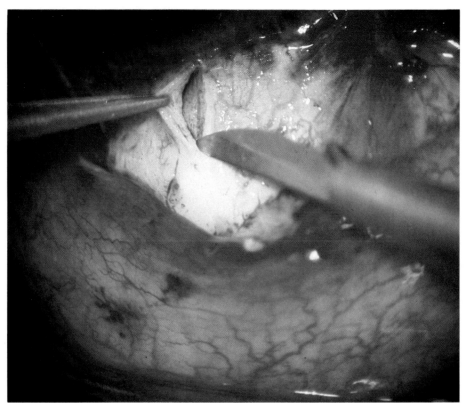

Figure 4.16. Technique for trabeculotomy (continued). A radial incision extending from the surgical limbus posteriorly for 3 mm is made in the sclera and dissected down until the landmarks of the deeper structures are just visible.

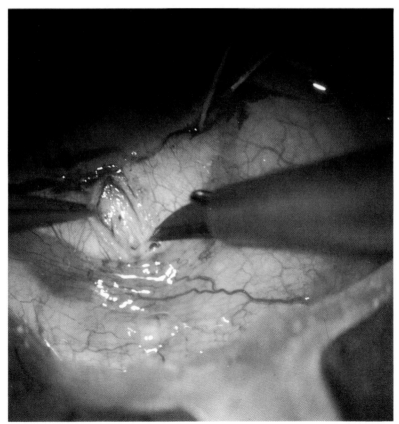

Figure 4.17. Technique for trabeculotomy (continued). The radial incision is undermined on each side at the level at which the deepest structures are just visible.

ing from the surgical limbus at the midpoint of the exposed sclera posteriorly for 3 mm (Fig. 4.16). Holding one edge of this incision with forceps and rotating it outward to allow greater visibility, the scleral incision is deepened until corneal and trabeculum tissue becomes visible in the depths of the anterior half of the incision (Fig. 4.17). At this point, the incision is undermined on each side to increase the surgical exposure (Fig. 4.18). Once the undermining has been completed, the surgeon has a view of the external surgical landmarks and can proceed to the next step, which is the dissection of the external wall of the canal of Schlemm. These surgical landmarks are well illustrated in Figures 4.18 and 4.19. From above is cornea, and looking downward the next structure is the surgical limbus. It is at the surgical limbus that the dissection commences. In the depths of the dissection, just below the surgical limbus, is transparent-looking tissue which represents deep corneal tissue. Look-

ing further downward in the illustration, the next structure below the transparent corneal tissue is a band of grayish, less transparent tissue which represents the trabecular band. Still looking downward, this trabecular band suddenly ceases and is replaced by white, dense, opaque scleral tissue. The junction of the lower limit of the trabecular band and the scleral tissue represents a landmark for the scleral spur, and it is in this area that the canal of Schlemm will be found. This point is in most eyes 2 to 2.5 mm behind the surgical limbus.

DISSECTION INTO CANAL
(15× MAGNIFICATION)

Having recognized these landmarks, the next step is to make a vertical incision using a microblade (e.g., a 75 Beaver blade) across the scleral spur at the junction of the lower margin of the trabeculum band and the scleral tissue (Fig. 4.18). This incision is carefully deepened until it is carried through the

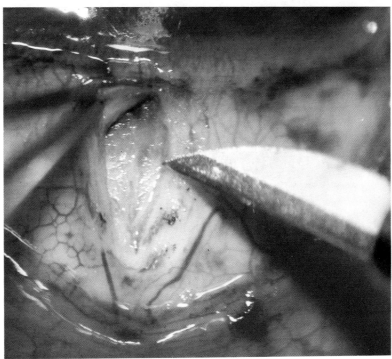

Figure 4.18. Technique for trabeculotomy (continued). Adequate exposure is obtained of the deeper layers in the sclera. The surgical landmarks are easily visible. Closest to the limbus is a blue-colored band of deep corneal lamellae, behind that is a narrower grayish-blue band which is trabecular meshwork and behind the trabecular meshwork is sclera. The junction of the posterior border of the trabecular band and the sclera is the external landmark for the scleral spur and the landmark for the canal of Schlemm. A radial incision is made, visible in the photograph, overlying the scleral spur in the deeper layers of the sclera in order to dissect down to the outer wall of the canal of Schlemm.

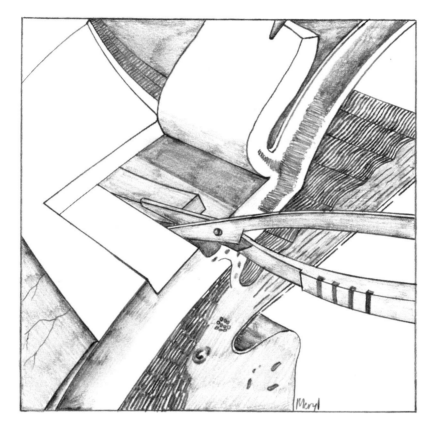

Figure 4.19. Technique for trabeculotomy (continued). A diagrammatic representation of the surgical landmarks in the deeper layers of the sclera as seen in Figure 4.18 and also surgical removal of 1.0 to 1.5 mm of the external wall of the canal of Schlemm. In this case, the dissection has been made under a 3-mm square one-third thickness scleral flap rather than using a radial incision (see technique for trabeculectomy, Chapter 8). The external surgical landmarks are indicated in the diagram. From above are shown the deep corneal lamellae, then a band which is the trabecular band and below the trabecular meshwork the sclera. The junction of the posterior border of the trabecular band and sclera is the landmark for the scleral spur and the canal of Schlemm. This is the position for making the radial incision to dissect the outer wall of Schlemm's canal shown in Figure 4.18.

A diagrammatic side section at the site of the radial incision illustrates the major tissue landmarks beneath the lamellar scleral flap. One blade of a Vannas scissor has been introduced into the canal, and dissection of the roof of the canal is begun.

external wall of Schlemm's canal, at which point there is a gush of aqueous and occasionally aqueous mixed with blood. The dissection is carefully continued through the external wall until the inner wall of the canal becomes visible. The inner wall is characteristically slightly pigmented and is composed of crisscrossing fibers (Figs. 4.20 and 4.21). Once this point is reached, one blade of Vannas scissors is passed into the canal through the opening in the external wall (Fig. 4.22) and a strip of the external wall of the canal is excised. In this way, the canal is opened for 1.0 to 1.5 mm circumferentially (Figs. 4.20 and 4.21). When introducing the blade of the Vannas scissors, it should enter the canal with ease and slide along the canal. If not, then a false passage is being produced and the external wall of the canal has not been adequately dissected.

INTRODUCTION OF TRABECULOTOMY PROBE (5× MAGNIFICATION)

A trabeculotomy probe of the design shown in Figure 4.23 is introduced. Other designs for a trabeculotomy probe are described (Della Porta, Lee Allan, Harms, Dobree). The lower blade has a diameter of 0.20 mm and fits into the canal; the upper blade runs over the limbus and, if kept resting on the cornea, ensures that the lower blade does not press downward through the inner wall of the canal or ride upward, creating a false passage. The two blades are separated by 1 mm. The shaft of the probe is divided into three segments so that the central third can be stabilized with the left hand, while the right hand rotates the upper and lower thirds around the central third, rotating the probe into the anterior chamber (Fig. 4.24). This method will avoid anterior or posterior movement of the

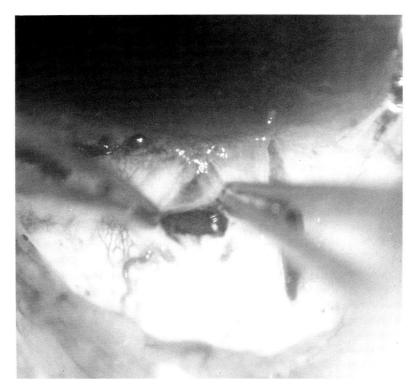

Figure 4.20.   Technique for trabeculotomy (continued). The radial incision made over the external landmark for the scleral spur, indicated in Figure 4.18, has been dissected through the external wall of Schlemm's canal and into the lumen of the canal. The roof of Schlemm's canal has been removed in the area that is surgically exposed within the radial scleral incision. In this photograph, one is looking directly at the lumen of the canal of Schlemm and the internal wall of the canal, which is characteristically darkly pigmented. Anterior to the canal one can see the blue-colored lamellae of cornea, and posterior to the canal is sclera. Adjacent to the section of the canal is another radial incision which was abandoned when the anterior chamber was accidentally entered. A major advantage of the radial incision, as opposed to dissecting a one-third or one-half thickness scleral flap, is that if anything goes wrong with the dissection another radial incision is easily made in an adjacent area of sclera without enlarging the conjunctival flap.

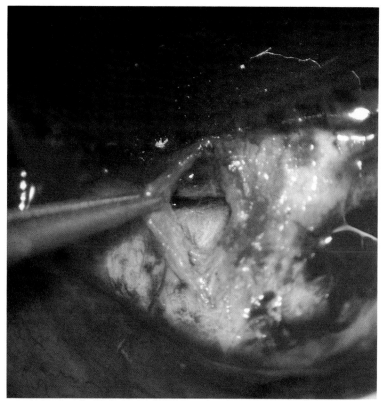

Figure 4.21. Technique for trabeculotomy (continued). Another view of the unroofed Schlemm's canal and the internal wall seen through a radial scleral incision.

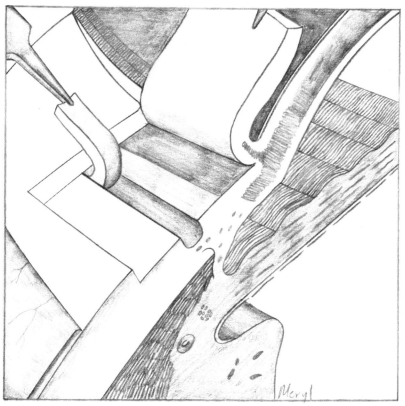

Figure 4.22. Technique for trabeculotomy (continued). Diagrammatic representation of unroofing the outer wall of the canal of Schlemm, in this case under a one-third thickness 3-mm wide scleral flap as opposed to a radial incision. The outer wall has been opened by a radial incision (Fig. 4.19). One blade of a Vannas scissor is introduced into the lumen of the canal through the radial incision, moved along the lumen and the outer wall of Schlemm's canal is dissected off for 1.0 to 1.5 mm.

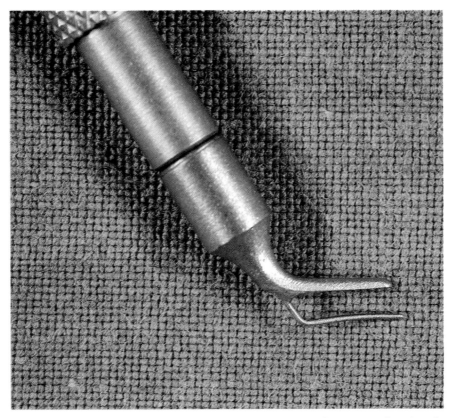

Figure 4.23. Technique for trabeculotomy (continued). Luntz trabeculotomy probe showing the 0.20-mm diameter probe used for entering the canal lumen. Separated by 1 mm is a thicker metal indicator which lies over the sclera and indicates the position of the probe when it is in the canal.

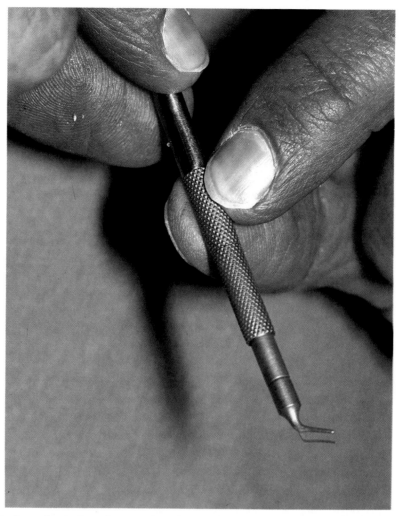

Figure 4.24. Technique for trabeculotomy (continued). Luntz trabeculotomy probe showing the break in the shaft which allows the probe to be held and controlled with the left hand while it is rotated into the anterior chamber by turning the shaft with the right hand. In this way, the left hand ensures that the probe remains in the same horizontal plane as it rotates and does not move downward into the iris or upward into the cornea. (Manufactured by Keeler, London, U.K.)

probe tip, avoiding iris trauma or disruption of corneal lamellae.

The probe is passed along the canal to the nasal side (Fig. 4.25) and rotated into the anterior chamber, thus opening the inner wall of the canal (Fig. 4.26). The same process is repeated on the other side, again rotating the probe into the anterior chamber. The probe is withdrawn, and, if the procedure has been adequately performed, a bridge of the inner wall of the canal of Schlemm remains intact across the area of canal that was unroofed. This bridge is composed of the inner wall of the canal and prevents the iris prolapsing into the surgical incision so that a peripheral iridectomy is not necessary. If the iris does prolapse into the incision, then a peripheral iridectomy should be performed.

If is very important that no force is used when introducing the probe into the canal, as this will create a false passage. If the probe does not slip easily down the canal, it implies that the probe is not properly in the canal due to inadequate dissection of all the fibers of the external wall. When this occurs, the probe is withdrawn and the dissection of the outer wall is continued using a sharp microblade until the surgeon is satisfied that all fibers of the outer wall are removed. Then it is tested by once more passing the probe down the canal.

During the procedure, the anterior chamber should be present at all times. As the probe passes into the anterior chamber, disrupting the inner wall of the canal, there is usually a little intracameral bleeding from the inner wall.

As the probe is swung from the canal into the

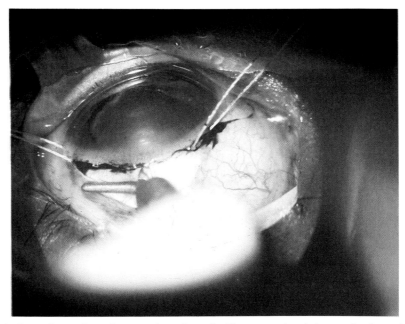

Figure 4.25. Technique for trabeculotomy (continued). Photograph of the probe introduced into the canal of Schlemm showing the guiding probe on the sclera.

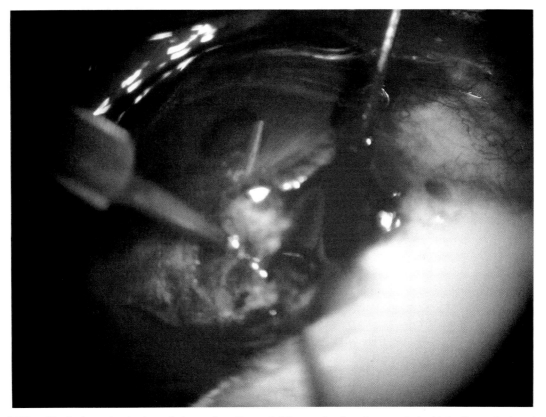

Figure 4.26. Technique for trabeculotomy (continued). The probe has been rotated into the anterior chamber and can be seen lying in the anterior chamber.

anterior chamber, the surgeon should carefully watch the iris for any movement. Movement of the iris implies that the probe is catching the iris surface, and this may result in an irido-dialysis. The probe should be immediately withdrawn without continuing its entry into the anterior chamber and then replaced, keeping the tip of the probe slightly anterior so that it does not rupture the inner wall prematurely. The cornea should also be carefully monitored to ensure that the probe is not ripping through the scleral tissue, cornea and Descemet's membrane. This is easy to detect because small air bubbles appear in the cornea as the probe progresses through the corneal lamellae. This occurs when the probe tip is in the sclera, and the probe should be repositioned, pushing the tip a little posteriorly.

The important points are that the probe should pass with ease along the canal and from the canal into the anterior chamber without use of force.

Some surgeons (Harms) prefer to do trabeculotomy under a lamellar scleral flap. This technique is described below under "Surgical Technique for Trabeculectomy-Trabeculotomy."

CLOSURE OF THE INCISION

Closure of the procedure is achieved with three virgin silk sutures in the scleral incision, conjunctival flap is rotated forward to the limbus and secured with one 10/0 suture at each edge.

POSTOPERATIVE MONITORING

Careful monitoring of the postoperative course is essential. The blood in the anterior chamber should absorb by the first or second postoperative day, the cornea remains clear and there is minimal iritis. An antibiotic steroid eyedrop can be used but should not be necessary for more than 3 to 4 days.

Six weeks postoperatively, the child is examined under anesthesia, and the intraocular pressure, corneal diameter and gonioscopic appearance of the angle are recorded. Gonioscopically, a cleft is visible at the site of the trabeculotomy, situated just anterior to the iris root in the position of the canal of Schlemm (Fig. 4.27). Pressure at the limbus with a gonioscope may result in a retrograde flow of blood along Schlemm's canal which escapes through the ruptured inner wall at its junction with intact inner wall. When this occurs, it is good evidence that the trabeculotomy is functional (Fig. 4.28).

When the result is satisfactory at the first examination, a second examination of intraocular pressure, corneal diameter and angle appearance is done 6 weeks later (3 months postoperative). If all is well, the next examination is done at 6 months and following this at yearly intervals.

The finding at any of these subsequent examinations of intraocular pressure raised above 18 mm Hg with corneal edema, or an increasing corneal diameter or an increase in the cup to disc ratio indicates the need to repeat the trabeculotomy procedure immediately at a different site.

CONGENITAL GLAUCOMA: COMPLICATIONS OF TRABECULOTOMY

There are very few complications associated with an adequately performed trabeculotomy. The senior author has operated on 110 eyes with C.I.J. glau-

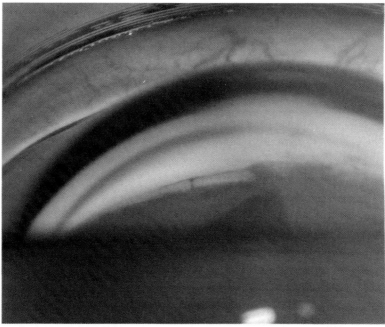

Figure 4.27. Technique for trabeculotomy (continued). Gonioscopy after trabeculotomy showing a cleft in the angle in the position of Schlemm's canal.

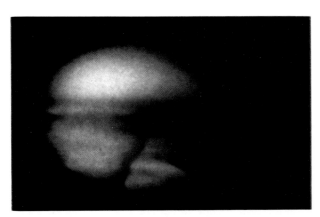

Figure 4.28. Technique for trabeculotomy (continued). Gonioscopy after trabeculotomy surgery. The slit lamp beam is placed at the junction of the ruptured inner wall of the canal of Schlemm and the intact inner wall. The ruptured inner wall is on the right-hand side of the photograph and the intact inner wall on the left-hand side. Pressure is applied to the limbal area, and blood can be seen trickling from the canal of Schlemm through the ruptured inner wall onto the iris surface.

coma by trabeculotomy with no significant complications. The major risks are:

1. Postoperative hyphema. It is usual for some bleeding to occur when the trabeculotomy probe ruptures the wall of the canal of Schlemm and enters the anterior chamber. Generally, this blood has absorbed by the day after surgery, or at the least within two days. Persistent bleeding occurs only if the iris root has been torn by the trabeculotomy probe and an irido-dialysis produced.

2. Traumatic irido-dialysis. This occurs if the trabeculotomy probe is inadvertently pushed through the inner wall of the canal of Schlemm, tangles the iris stroma and tears the iris base off the ciliary body as the probe is swept into the anterior chamber. This is easily avoided by watching the iris surface as the probe is slowly swept from the canal into the anterior chamber. If there is any movement of the iris surface, then the probe should be withdrawn and re-inserted. Tearing the iris root results in a large hyphema and the possibility of secondary glaucoma. One can wait for the hyphema to absorb with time if the intraocular pressure remains normal. When secondary glaucoma does occur and cannot be medically controlled, then a paracentesis should be done and the hyphema evacuated.

3. Tearing of Descemet's membrane or corneal stroma. This occurs if the trabeculotomy probe creates a false passage through the anterior wall of the canal into the sclera, or if the anterior wall of the canal is not adequately dissected and a false passage is made into the sclera. If this occurs there is undue resistance to passage of the probe, the cornea buckles and small air bubbles form between the corneal lamellae in front of the probe. The probe should be withdrawn, the outer wall of the canal dissected into the canal lumen and the probe re-inserted.

4. Formation of a conjunctival bleb. Conjunctival bleb formation occurs if the scleral wound is not adequately sutured at the end of the procedure. This did not occur in any of the 110 cases in this series.

5. Staphyloma of the sclera is another complication of inadequate suturing of the scleral incision.

6. Failure to control intraocular pressure. The causes for failure are discussed under "Management of C.I.J. Glaucoma and the Prognosis for Surgery." When the operation fails to control intraocular pressure, it can be repeated a maximum of three times. With persistent failure, a trabeculectomy should be done.

7. Failure to find the canal of Schlemm. Absence of the canal of Schlemm is a rare anomaly. The canal is consistently located 2 mm behind the limbus unless the angle has a cicatricial component. In the latter case, the canal is found closer to the limbus. In some eyes, the canal is collapsed and difficult to identify. In such difficult cases, careful dissection within the plane of the trabecular tissue from the limbus posteriorly for 2.5 mm will usually locate the canal somewhere within this area. Even when the canal is collapsed, the inner wall can be identified by its characteristic appearance of pigmented, crisscrossing trabecular fibers.

GONIOTOMY

Goniotomy is an alternative procedure to trabeculotomy. It is a more difficult technique than trabeculotomy and not advised unless one is well trained in this technique. The technique for goniotomy has been well described by several authors, particularly Barkan (1942).

Trabeculotomy is the preferred operation for the reasons stated at the beginning of this chapter.

SURGICAL TECHNIQUE FOR TRABECULECTOMY-TRABECULOTOMY

The technique of trabeculectomy is described in detail in Chapter 8, and only an outline of the surgical technique is offered here.

A 7-mm fornix-based conjunctival flap is raised in the superior limbus. This is reflected back to expose sclera with sufficient space to outline with

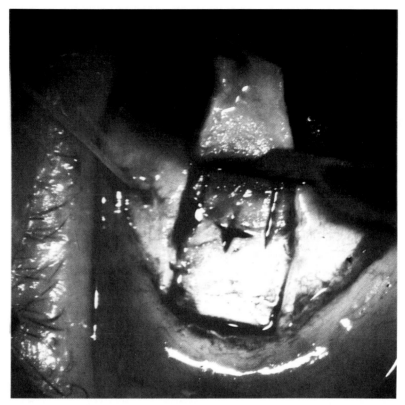

Figure 4.29. Technique for combined trabeculectomy-trabeculotomy. Photograph of the exposure for trabeculectomy-trabeculotomy. A 7-mm wide fornix-based conjunctival flap is reflected backward. A 3 mm × 3 mm scleral flap of one-third thickness has been raised and hinged forward over the cornea. (See surgical techniques for trabeculectomy, Chapter 8). In the bed of this dissection, one can recognize the surgical landmarks. A 2 mm × 2 mm flap is outlined extending from cornea at the base of the scleral flap backward by two radial incisions to the scleral spur. A radial dissection across the external landmarks for the scleral spur is made in the center of this deep bed to dissect down to the outer wall of Schlemm's canal. The operation for trabeculotomy and trabeculectomy then continues in the manner described in the text (for trabeculectomy, see Chapter 8).

cautery a 3 mm × 3 mm scleral flap. A one-third thickness scleral flap hinged at the limbus is raised and rotated anteriorly onto the cornea. The external surgical landmarks are now visible, viz. deep corneal tissue anteriorly, a band of trabecular tissue behind this and sclera behind the trabecular band.

Following the technique for trabeculectomy described in Chapter 8, a 2 mm × 2 mm block is outlined in the deep corneal and trabecular tissue at the base of the scleral flap, extending posteriorly to the scleral spur which is at the junction of the posterior margin of the trabecular band and the scleral tissue. This block is incised to the deep layers without entering the anterior chamber (Fig. 4.29).

A radial incision is cut across the trabecular band and across the scleral spur (Fig. 4.29) and dissected downward until the canal of Schlemm is identified. The canal is situated 2 mm behind the surgical limbus and at the external landmark for the scleral spur (see Chapter 8). Once the outer wall of the canal is dissected into its lumen, a small sinusotomy (removal of the outer wall of the canal) is made on each side of the radial incision with Vannas scissors, a trabeculotomy probe is inserted and a trabeculotomy is performed on each side of the radial incision. At completion of the trabeculotomy, the anterior chamber should still be intact. Attention is now directed to the 2 mm × 2 mm square of corneal and trabecular tissue previously outlined, and the operation for trabeculectomy is completed as described in Chapter 8. If trabeculectomy alone is chosen, then the description of this operation in Chapter 8 is followed.

OTHER SURGICAL PROCEDURES FOR C.I.J. GLAUCOMA

Other filtration operations—for example, Elliot's trephine operation, iridencleisis, posterior sclerectomy—have been tried in eyes with C.I.J. glaucoma that do not respond well to trabeculotomy or are unlikely to respond well. These procedures have a higher risk of complications than trabeculectomy, and there is no documented evidence of a higher success rate than with trabeculectomy. For this reason, trabeculectomy remains the filtration operation of choice.

PLASTIC FILTRATION DEVICES

These devices are reserved for those eyes refractory to surgery in which one or more trabeculotomies and trabeculectomies have failed to control the intraocular pressure. There are a number of alternatives:

1. Simple setons placed through the sclera just posterior to the limbus. These are uniformly unsuccessful in the long run.

2. Krupin-Denver valve prosthesis, manufactured by Storz. Essentially, these are plastic setons with a pressure-sensitive valve which controls the flow of aqueous through the seton. There is only a limited experience with this technique, and it has not been encouraging.

3. The draining tube reported by Molteno and Luntz (1969) and subsequently further improved by Molteno (1980) has been used with encouraging results for up to 15 years in congenital glaucoma refractory to other drainage operations. This is the method favored by the authors. The surgical technique is described in detail in Chapter 11.

CYCLOCRYOTHERAPY

Cyclocryotherapy is indicated if all other surgical procedures have failed. The surgical method is described in detail in Chapter 8.

VISUAL REHABILITATION FOLLOWING CONTROL OF INTRAOCULAR PRESSURE

Unfortunately, control of the intraocular pressure in a child with C.I.J. glaucoma is only the first step in the management of the disease. The child with C.I.J. glaucoma suffers significant disturbance during the critical developmental phase of his or her visual abilities. As a result, even after control of intraocular pressure, patients with C.I.J. glaucoma are usually amblyopic and have little or no binocular vision. Following successful surgery, these children need a protracted course of orthoptics to rehabilitate vision. The principles involved are:

1. Adequate refraction and optical correction with spectacles or contact lenses.

2. Patching the "good" eye in an attempt to reverse the amblyopia.

3. Alternate patching once amblyopia has been reversed.

4. Orthoptic treatment to promote binocular fusion.

The visual rehabilitation outlined above will need close cooperation between ophthalmologist, orthoptist and parents.

Section 2

ADULT ONSET GLAUCOMAS

Maurice H. Luntz, M.D.

Professor of Ophthalmology
Mt. Sinai School of Medicine
Director of Ophthalmology
Beth Israel Medical Center

Consultant
Manhattan Eye, Ear, & Throat Hospital
New York, New York

and

Raymond Harrison, M.D.

Attending Surgeon and Director
Glaucoma Service
Manhattan Eye, Ear & Throat Hospital
New York, New York

Chapter 5

PREOPERATIVE PREPARATION AND ANESTHESIA FOR GLAUCOMA SURGERY

Adequate preoperative evaluation of the patient's general medical condition is of great importance. A proper medical history is mandatory. A general physical examination is essential; and basic laboratory investigations should be routinely required, consisting of a complete blood count, chemistries profile including electrolytes and prothrombin time, urinalysis, electrocardiogram and chest x-ray (in patients over 40). Control of high blood pressure and diabetes and correction of hypokalemia in patients taking carbonic anhydrase inhibitors are commonly needed before surgery. Preoperative osmotherapy may be contraindicated in patients with angina. Use of long acting cholinesterase inhibitors is important information for the anesthesiologist if succinylcholine use is anticipated. Herpetic disease may preclude the use of general anesthesia. These are but a few examples of the value of careful preoperative medical scrutiny.

ANESTHESIA

Either local or general anesthesia may be acceptable, depending on the choice of the surgeon and the patient. The patient's general medical status and temperament must be considered. The tendency is toward the use of local anesthesia.

Local Anesthesia

The choice of premedication for local anesthetic and the drugs for the local block are individual to each surgeon. There are a few important principles:

1. Sedative and hypnotic drugs used in the premedication should be used sparingly because the patient's cerebration and respiration should not be excessively depressed.

2. A Van Lint block of upper and lower eyelids is generally sufficient to produce lid akinesia for the duration of the surgery.

3. A mixture of a short acting local anesthesic (for example, Xylocaine 1.5%) with a long acting local anesthetic (for example, Marcaine 0.5%) is very effective.

4. A retrobulbar injection is used to anesthetize the iris for the iridectomy. Full akinesia of extraocular muscles is not necessary if the patient is phakic and lens extraction is not being performed. For this reason, injection of 1 cc of a short acting retrobulbar anesthetic (for example, Xylocaine 1.5%) is sufficient.

5. Conjunctival anesthesia can be achieved by the use of topical tetracaine drops. Subconjunctival injection of local anesthetic is not necessary, although it may aid in the dissection of a conjunctival flap.

General Anesthesia

General anesthesia is preferred in those patients requiring combined cataract surgery and glaucoma surgery and in aphakic patients requiring glaucoma surgery. Another relative indication for general anesthesia is for those patients who have cardiac or vascular disease and may be at risk of cardiac complications during surgery. The advantage is that the patient is on a full life support system in case of such complications. General anesthesia from the surgeon's viewpoint assures a quiet, immobile patient with full akinesia of the extraocular muscles. The preferred general anesthesia is Pentothal and succinylcholine induction given intravenously, followed by intubation, muscle paralysis and a closed circuit breathing system with assisted respiration. The anesthetist should be familiar with the requirements of anesthesia for eye surgery and familiar with the surgery itself.

PREOPERATIVE PREPARATION

Once the patient is anesthetized, the operative field is prepared using antiseptics. The choice of antiseptics is an individual one, but certain principles are important:

1. Both eyes should be cleaned and "prepped." This ensures that the surgeon or assistant will not touch potentially septic areas during draping the patient and preparing the operative area. The cleansing of the skin should begin with a routine cleaning wash using saline, followed by a solution containing a detergent or soap, followed by the application of an antiseptic solution (for example, Betadine) and then removal of all the solutions from the area with alcohol. Both eyes are anesthetized with a topical anesthetic before the application of antiseptic solutions, and the patient is instructed to keep the eyes closed if local anesthesia is being used.

After suitably cleansing the operative field, the patient is draped with sterile towels, exposing the eye to be operated on. The next step is to apply a sterile plastic dressing. The plastic drape (Steridrape) should be applied in such a way that it covers the skin of the eyelid and the eyelashes, leaving only the conjunctival surface of the globe exposed. Exposure of the globe can then be achieved by the use of a Barraquer wire speculum or Pierse adjustable speculum. These are applied after the eyelids have been cleaned and before the drapes and Steridrape are applied. They give excellent exposure with minimum pressure on the globe. The exposed eye is irrigated with an antibiotic solution (e.g., Neosporin) before commencement of surgery.

Chapter 6

SELECTION OF SURGICAL PROCEDURE

SELECTING THE BEST SUITED OPERATION

It is important to select the operative procedure most likely to succeed for a particular problem. No single operative procedure will effectively control intraocular pressure in all types of glaucoma or in every individual. The operations that we generally prefer are trabeculotomy, peripheral iridectomy, peripheral laser iridotomy, subscleral trabeculectomy, subscleral Scheie (subscleral thermosclerostomy, see Chapter 8), laser trabeculoplasty (trabecular retraction) and cyclocryotherapy. Laser "iridostomy" is a more appropriate term than laser iridotomy or iridectomy.

In order to select the surgical procedure that will give the best results in any given case of glaucoma, two major parameters that require evaluation are the intraocular pressure and gonioscopy. The results of surgery in glaucoma will always correlate well with these two parameters.

Developmental Angle Anomalies (Trabeculotomy or Trabeculectomy)

These anomalies presumably obstruct the trabecular tissue, resulting in increased intraocular pressure. They are present at birth, but glaucoma may present either at or soon after birth (congenital glaucoma) or later (infantile glaucoma or juvenile glaucoma) or even in later adult life. Juvenile glaucoma may be due to either the late onset of glaucoma from a developmental angle anomaly (recognized gonioscopically) or early onset open angle glaucoma in which the angle appears normal and is open (see Section 1).

INDICATIONS FOR SURGERY

Surgery is always the treatment of choice as these patients do not do well with long term medical therapy. The best surgical result with the least traumatic intervention is either trabeculotomy, if the angle anomaly is a presumed mesodermal anomaly (irrespective of the age of onset), or trabeculectomy, if the angle anomaly is a cicatricial process in the angle or an irido-corneal dysgenesis (see Section 1). In juvenile glaucoma due to a mesodermal angle anomaly, the operation of choice is trabeculotomy, but if due to open angle glaucoma, the surgical management follows the same principles as described for open angle glaucoma.

Closed Angle (Peripheral Iridectomy or Subscleral Scheie)

Angle closure glaucoma is best treated surgically and with few exceptions does well with peripheral iridectomy, which is the operation of choice. The exceptions are those cases in which, following attempted reversal of an acute angle closure attack, the angle remains more than 75% closed even with indentation gonioscopy and/or the intraocular pressure remains over 45 mm Hg on full medication. The prognosis for peripheral iridectomy is poor in these cases (a success rate of only 43%) (Luntz, 1969), and these patients can be spared a second surgical procedure by doing a subscleral Scheie operation initially. If the intraocular pressure at operation is high, a posterior sclerotomy with removal of fluid vitreous will decompress the eye before doing the subscleral Scheie.

Trabeculectomy is successful in controlling intraocular pressure in only 60 to 65% of these eyes, whereas with the subscleral Scheie, the success rate is 80% or better. The added postoperative risks of the Scheie operation are acceptable because of the significantly higher success rate.

INDENTATION GONIOSCOPY

Indentation gonioscopy (Forbes) is a useful diagnostic technique to determine whether an angle which appears to be closed is sealed by peripheral synechiae, or whether the iris is merely in contact with the posterior corneal surface and can be opened. One method is to use the four-mirror Zeiss goniolens. This is placed on the eye and then pushed directly inward, flattening the cornea and increasing intracameral pressure, thus forcibly opening the angle if there are no permanent peripheral anterior synechiae. Another method is to use a one- or two-mirror Goldmann gonioscope with a small flange. This is placed on the cornea in the usual manner and the angle visualized. If the angle appears to be closed, the gonioscope is tilted to put pressure on the limbus, a maneuver which increases the aqueous pressure in the anterior chamber, thereby forcing open the angle on the opposite side if it is not sealed by synechiae. Thus, if one is looking through the superior mirror at the inferior angle, pressure is applied superiorly by tilting the upper part of the gonioscope into the globe, and the inferior angle will open if it is not sealed. The same maneuver can be repeated around the circumference of the limbus, enabling one accurately to document areas of the angle that are permanently closed and those that appear to be closed but are in fact open.

In chronic angle closure where appositional closure exists, in contradistinction to peripheral anterior synechiae, Chandler's procedure of anterior chamber deepening was valuable when surgical iridectomy was more frequently done. With the patient prepared for surgery, a small Wheeler knife paracentesis is preferred to permit drainage of aqueous from both the anterior and posterior chambers. The anterior chamber is then deepened with saline injected via the corneal stab incision. This maneuver will open areas of appositional closure. The Koeppe gonioscopy lens should be used in this procedure to evaluate the circumferential extent of peripheral anterior synechiae. An inexperienced surgeon doing this procedure may find it difficult to interpret. Too much fluid injected into the anterior chamber may cause the lens to subluxate. Laser peripheral iridectomy has rendered this maneuver obsolete.

MANAGEMENT OF THE FELLOW (SECOND) EYE IN A PATIENT WITH PRIMARY ANGLE CLOSURE GLAUCOMA

It is generally agreed that the fellow (second) eye in a patient who has suffered a typical acute attack of unilateral primary angle closure glaucoma will have an anterior chamber of approximately equal narrowness to the involved eye and is exposed to a high risk of an acute angle closure attack. This observation was made by Bain in 1957 and later confirmed by Lowe. Bain, following 200 cases of acute unilateral closed angle glaucoma, showed that 53% of fellow (second) eyes that were on miotic treatment developed acute attacks in an average period of 4.25 years and of those fellow (second) eyes that were untreated, 78% had an acute attack or prodromal symptoms. He suggested that prophylactic peripheral iridectomy is a safer protection against trouble than miotic therapy. As a result of these observations, it has become routine to perform a prophylactic peripheral iridectomy in fellow (second) eyes of patients with unilateral primary angle closure glaucoma.

For the past 10 years, prior to the advent of the laser, we have done prophylactic "invasive" surgery in the fellow (second) eye only in those patients who have a definite previous history or symptoms of acute episodes of angle closure or a positive dark room test in the second eye. The dark room provocative test is of major importance in considering treatment for angle closure glaucoma (Luntz, 1981).

When these above criteria are absent, it is not necessary to treat the fellow (second) eye, but careful re-evaluation of the history and dark room test is repeated approximately every 4 months. The patient must be made familiar with the symptoms of an angle closure episode and must be told to report immediately if any of these symptoms occur.

Using these criteria in 65 fellow (second) eyes, 45 required prophylactic peripheral iridectomy after the iridectomy on the first eye. The remaining 20 were followed. Seven developed positive criteria but without an acute attack and had peripheral iridectomy. The 13 remaining eyes have been followed for over 10 years, and of these only 1 (7%) developed an acute attack, which was successfully treated with peripheral iridectomy, representing 1 false negative in 65 eyes (1.5%) (Luntz, 1981). With the high level of safety of laser iridotomy it has now become more acceptable to do routine laser iridotomy on the "fellow" (second) eye.

Open Angle Glaucoma

INDICATIONS FOR SURGERY IN OPEN ANGLE GLAUCOMA

Intolerance of Medication

Some patients cannot tolerate medication and require surgery for adequate control. For example, asthmatics may not tolerate Timoptic or echothiophate, young myopes and elderly patients with incipient cataracts may not tolerate miotics and patients commonly develop side effects with carbonic anhydrase inhibitors. The latter should not be used indefinitely in younger patients.

Failure to Control the Disease Adequately

1. Progressive loss of visual field despite good compliance with medication and good tolerance.

2. Intraocular pressures consistently above 35 to 40 mm Hg on maximal medical treatment without progression of field loss.

3. Severe visual field deficit and intraocular pressure at all times over 15 mm Hg on full medication. Severe visual field deficit implies:
   a. "Tubular" field.
   b. Field loss extending into the 10 degree isopter at any point.
   c. History of rapid extension of the visual field defect into fixation in the other eye (first eye) at similar intraocular pressure levels.

4. Patients with ocular hypertension, over age 65 years and intraocular pressure over 26 mm Hg on full medication (danger of retinal venous occlusion) (Luntz and Schenker, 1980).

5. Patients with ocular hypertension and intraocular pressures rising to over 40 mm Hg on full medication.

6. Documented progressive enlargement of optic disc cup to a cup to disc ratio of 0.6 to 0.7, especially in the vertical axis.

7. Myopes with large, saucer-shaped optic nerve heads and intraocular pressures rising to over 30 mm Hg.

Secondary Glaucoma: Indications for Surgery

Surgical intervention is indicated when full medical treatment of the primary disease has failed to overcome resistance to aqueous flow at the pupil or the angle. Uveitis is the commonest underlying disease process. When extensive peripheral anterior synechiae and angle damage have occurred, a trabeculectomy or subscleral Scheie is necessary. Seclusio pupillae can be abolished simply by peripheral iridectomy (surgical or laser) if the iris plane is bowed. Peripheral iridectomy and dissecting free the pupil or sector iridectomy is necessary if there is very extensive iris-lens adhesion. Transfixation of the iris is no longer advocated. Subluxation of the lens can lead to pupillary block. Mydriasis may break the block, but when this fails peripheral iridectomy (iridotomy, iridostomy) should be carried out. A cataractous lens should be extracted in the standard manner with peripheral iridectomy.

LASER TRABECULAR SURGERY

Argon laser trabecular surgery (trabeculoplasty) will lower intraocular pressure an average of 10 mm Hg in 80% of treated eyes with as large a fall as 25 mm Hg (personal experience). It can be used only if the angle is open and the scleral spur is clearly visualized. A narrow angle can often be opened adequately for this procedure by gonioplasty (see Chapter 8) or by laser peripheral iridectomy in cases of mixed glaucoma. When laser trabecular surgery has failed, then subscleral trabeculectomy or subscleral Scheie is advised.

The complications of laser trabecular surgery are, on the whole, minimal: pigment dispersion within the anterior chamber, iritis, superficial corneal burns and, in about 20% of treated eyes, a marked rise in intraocular pressure immediately after treatment and lasting up to approximately 5 days. The latter complication can lead to loss of fixation in an eye with advanced glaucoma and a very compromised visual field. Consequently, some surgeons consider laser trabecular surgery to be contraindicated in advanced glaucoma. Laser trabecular surgery, when adequately monitored, carries only minimal risk and should be considered as the first surgical choice in open angle glaucoma.

TRABECULECTOMY OR SCHEIE

The operation of choice will depend on the level of intraocular pressure with maximum well tolerated medication, which is also an indication of the amount of functioning trabecular meshwork available.

Trabeculectomy

It is important to recognize that trabeculectomy is not the best operation in every case of open angle glaucoma. Trabeculectomy is not as efficient a filtering procedure as a Scheie, but it is much safer if the lamellar scleral flap is sutured into place. The trabeculectomy operation will, on average, reduce intraocular pressure by 16 mm Hg, with a range of 12 to 25 mm Hg. Therefore, in selecting the surgical procedure for open angle glaucoma, note should be taken of the pressure-lowering effect that is required. This will depend on the intraocular pressure the patient maintains on maximally effective and well tolerated medication, as well as the final intraocular pressure that is desired. For example, if a patient has a good visual field and an average intraocular pressure on full medication of 35 mm Hg, then trabeculectomy is a suitable procedure because the anticipated postoperative intraocular pressure will average below 20 mm Hg. With similar pressures and a visual field which is approaching fixation, then a greater pressure-reducing effect is required, and subscleral Scheie is the procedure of choice.

Subscleral Scheie

Subscleral Scheie is used in eyes with intraocular pressure exceeding 45 mm Hg on full medication and/or eyes in which 75% or more of the circumference of the angle is closed by permanent synechiae as demonstrated with indentation gonioscopy. This includes most eyes with secondary glaucoma. Whereas trabeculectomy will control intraocular pressure in approximately 60 to 65% of these eyes, the subscleral Scheie is 80% or more effective (Luntz, 1981). The operation, however, carries a higher risk of postoperative complications, particularly shallow or flat anterior chamber, hypotony, malignant glaucoma and cataract. In properly selected cases, these additional risks are justified by the superior pressure control achieved.

Indications for Subscleral Trabeculectomy

1. Angle closure glaucoma with less than 75% of the angle closed by peripheral anterior synechiae.

2. Adult open angle glaucoma. Intraocular pressure on full medication lower than 40 mm Hg if the visual field is not severely affected, but 30 mm Hg or lower if the field is severely affected.

3. Pigmentary glaucoma.

4. Aniridia.

5. Pseudocapsular exfoliation. Eyes with pseudocapsular exfoliation often have very high intraocular pressures even with full medication. These do remarkably well with trabeculectomy and are an exception to the previously described limitations of the operation.

6. Open angle glaucoma in an aphakic patient. The prognosis must always be guarded in aphakia, and an anterior vitrectomy must be combined with the trabeculectomy unless the vitreous face is well formed and well behind the pupil. When in doubt, an anterior vitrectomy should be done.

7. Rubeosis iridis; essential iris atrophy; Chandler's syndrome. These are included in this category although they have a poorer prognosis with either laser trabeculoplasty, trabeculectomy (approxi-

mately 50% success rate) or subscleral Scheie. They do as well, however, with trabeculectomy as with more extensive filtration surgery, including valves or setons; for this reason, trabeculectomy is the initial operation of choice. This may be preceded by laser treatment of vessels in the angle and iris root.

Indications for Subscleral Scheie

We use the following guidelines as indications for the subscleral Scheie operation. Intraocular pressure on full medication in excess of 40 mm Hg with visual field defects outside the 10 degree isopter. When the visual field is more severely contracted (within the 10 degree isopter), this operation is indicated if intraocular pressure exceeds 30 mm Hg. There are also other situations in which this operation is indicated:

1. Young adult patients.

2. Previous failed trabeculectomy.

3. Low tension glaucoma if laser trabeculoplasty and trabeculectomy have failed. When these measures have failed in one eye, the fellow eye should be subjected to a subscleral Scheie as the first procedure of choice.

When the choice of procedure is in doubt, and particularly if the visual field is severely compromised, then trabeculectomy is preferred as the operation with fewer serious postoperative complications.

LOW TENSION GLAUCOMA

Role of Glaucoma Surgery in Progressive Low Tension Glaucoma

The question as to whether reducing intraocular pressure to very low levels, e.g., below 10 mm Hg, will arrest this disease cannot be answered in the individual case except in retrospect. There may be no alternative modality of therapy to offer the patient. It is our practice in these dire circumstances to advise an operation in one eye—the one with the more advanced visual loss. Laser trabecular surgery or a standard subscleral trabeculectomy is advocated. There is no virtue in choosing a full thickness filtering operation as a first procedure, unless the former measures have failed in the fellow eye.

Chapter 7

ANGLE CLOSURE GLAUCOMA

SURGICAL TREATMENT FOR ANGLE CLOSURE GLAUCOMA

In 1857, the German ophthalmologist Albrecht von Graefe announced at the first International Congress of Ophthalmology held in Brussels that he had discovered a surgical cure for acute glaucoma. This involved a sector iridectomy which he observed to effect a long-lasting cure. This discovery represented a major milestone in the history of ophthalmic surgery. Before von Graefe's discovery, acute glaucoma had been a blinding disease treated by leeches and venesection. Von Graefe had observed the hypotensive effect of a sector iridectomy performed for corneal staphyloma, and this led him to try it for acute glaucoma. It was not until 1920 that E. J. Curran, an American, noted that angle closure glaucoma was associated with pupil block and suggested that peripheral iridectomy was as effective in curing acute glaucoma as sector iridectomy. This has remained until recently the specific surgical treatment, but today the increased use of the argon laser to create a hole in the iris (laser iridotomy, iridectomy, iridostomy) has largely replaced surgical iridectomy in the United States.

SURGICAL TECHNIQUES FOR PERIPHERAL IRIDECTOMY OR IRIDOTOMY FOR ANGLE CLOSURE GLAUCOMA

Mechanism of Action

Peripheral iridectomy is a safe surgical procedure and highly successful in properly selected cases of angle closure glaucoma (see Chapter 6, "Selection of Surgical Procedure"). The objective is to create an opening for unhampered aqueous flow from the posterior to the anterior chamber, reducing the pressure buildup in the posterior chamber, thereby allowing the iris to fall backward and opening the angle. It is unnecessary to make the opening in the iris either basal or sector as long as aqueous can flow freely through it.

The equalization of pressure between the posterior and anterior chambers following iridectomy will separate iris from posterior corneal surface if the apposition has not become permanent. Attachments, resulting from long-standing occlusion of the angle, may become permanently scarred. At first this occurs intermittently in the angle, particularly if carbonic anhydrase inhibitors are used for any length of time to control an acute attack. The effect of the iridectomy on these attachments is to open localized areas of the angle where the closure is not permanent. The angle might only open adjacent to the iridectomy. This is due to loculation of the aqueous behind the iris as a result of widespread scar formation in the angle limiting the free flow of aqueous. In these long-standing cases, it is useful to do two peripheral iridectomies, one in each of the superior quadrants, because this may reach more than one locule of aqueous and open more of the angle than would only one iridectomy. Nevertheless, even in the above situation, one iridectomy, by equalizing anterior and posterior chamber pressures, will prevent further acute angle closure attacks. Any residual ocular hypertension after peripheral iridectomy is then due to either chronic angle closure or an open angle mechanism (primary or secondary).

SURGICAL TECHNIQUE

Incision

The operation is preferably performed through a corneal incision leaving the conjunctiva unmolested. A 3 mm long incision is made in the cornea just anterior to the limbus and at the anterior edge of the limbal corneal vessels.

The incision is best sited in the upper nasal quadrant using a #75 Beaver microblade. The corneal stroma is dissected down to Descemet's membrane. At this point, the scleral side of the incision is grasped with Hoskin #28 forceps (Keeler) and,

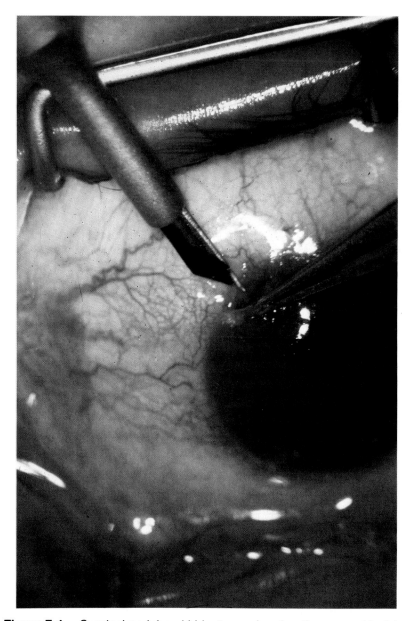

Figure 7.1. Surgical peripheral iridectomy showing the corneal incision.

keeping the cornea pulled slightly upward and away from the iris, the anterior chamber can be entered with the knife over the full 3-mm length of the incision. An operating microscope should be used at 10× magnification and with focal illumination (Fig. 7.1).

Iridectomy

Once the anterior chamber is entered, pressure is applied on the scleral side of the incision with a flat iris spatula in an attempt to prolapse the iris into the incision, in which case it is pulled through the incision using a #28 Hoskin forceps. When the iris does not prolapse into the incision, the forceps is carefully introduced into the anterior chamber using 10× magnification for good visualization of the iris surface. The iris is grasped with the forceps held in the left hand and pulled into the incision. The iris is then grasped at a point closer to the pupil with a second #28 Hoskin forceps held in the right hand and pulled out of the incision (Fig. 7.2). Failure to hold the iris nearer the pupil before pulling it through the incision may result in tearing the iris base, irido-dialysis and intraocular bleeding.

With the iris exteriorized, the surgeon ensures that both the stromal and pigment layer are held

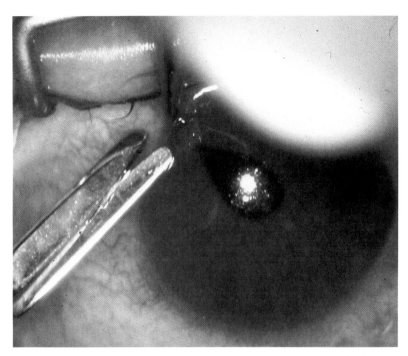

Figure 7.2.   Surgical peripheral iridectomy showing the iris pulled through the corneal incision.

in the forceps (pigment layer is usually easily visible through the iris stroma). Using a DeWecker scissor and cutting parallel to the limbus, the portion of the iris held in the forceps is removed. A peripheral iridectomy results at the junction of the outer and middle third of the iris surface. This is the ideal position for the peripheral iridectomy because the major iris vessels are avoided.

Return of the Iris to Anterior Chamber

In most cases, the iris once released will slip back through the incision into the anterior chamber, and the peripheral iridectomy can be visualized through the cornea. In the event iris becomes incarcerated in the incision, pressure on the scleral side of the incision with a flat iris spatula will generally dislodge it. Failing that, the cornea is stroked with an iris spatula from the center of the cornea upward to the limbus. When iris still remains incarcerated in the incision, the two edges of the incision are held apart and a jet of balanced salt solution directed into the incision will dislodge it.

Once the iris is back in the anterior chamber, the surgeon should ascertain that the iridectomy includes the pigment layer by demonstrating a red reflex through the iridectomy with retro-illumination using the slit beam microscope light.

Suturing the Incision

One 10-0 nylon suture is placed across the center of the corneal incision at full corneal depth, tied so as to provide good apposition but not too tightly. The suture is cut on the knot which is buried on the corneal side of the incision (Fig. 7.3). There is no necessity to reform the anterior chamber, as it is not lost during the procedure.

Subconjunctival injection of antibiotics and steroids is unnecessary. An antibiotic-steroid combination is used for a few days postoperatively. The suture can be left indefinitely or removed after 3 months. Suture-induced astigmatism is minimal because of the small size of the incision. There is minimal postoperative uveitis or discomfort.

RESULTS

Peripheral iridectomy is the most satisfying surgical procedure. When meticulous surgical technique is used a patent iridectomy is always obtained, and this will cure over 80% of primary angle closure glaucoma (Luntz, 1969). Late cataract formation is the commonest complication. Other complications are exceptionally rare but include wound leak, iritis, hyphema, malignant glaucoma and endophthalmitis.

Failure to excise the pigment layer of the iris will

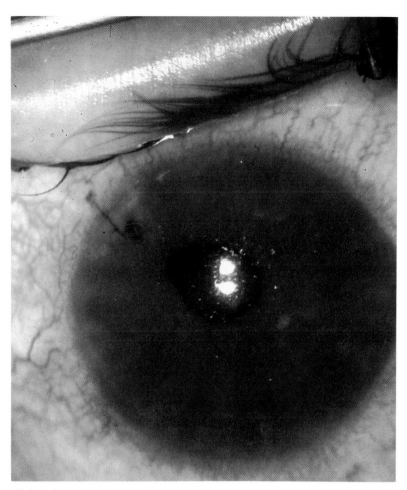

Figure 7.3.   Surgical peripheral iridectomy, the incision sutured with 10-0 nylon.

result in a nonfunctioning iridectomy. This is readily corrected using bursts of an argon laser set at 50 μ, 0.5 watt power and 0.2 second exposure, which will vaporize the pigment layer.

PERIPHERAL IRIDECTOMY (ALTERNATIVE TECHNIQUE) (RH)

A conjunctival flap including Tenon's fascia is made 4 mm from cornea and 5 mm in length. Incision into the anterior chamber is made with a diamond knife or razor knife or, if the surgeon prefers, the less sharp Bard Parker #15 blade. The latter is safer when peripheral anterior synechiae are present. The incision line is in the mid-limbal position. A "knuckle" of iris is prolapsed by gentle pressure on the posterior lip. Full thickness iridectomy is performed by DeWecker scissors applied radially, the iris being grasped with Bonn forceps. Loose iris pigment is irrigated away. A single suture of 10.0 nylon is usually adequate to close the incision, which should be tested for watertight closure by pressing with the tip of a fine forceps. The

conjunctival flap is closed with a short continuous 6-0 plain catgut suture. The anterior chamber is usually not lost but must be seen to be formed before allowing the patient to leave the operating room table. A drop of Cyclogyl 2% is instilled after irrigating the globe with chloramphenicol solution. Erythromycin ophthalmic ointment is applied to the closed lid margins, and an oval eye pad and metal shield are taped in position. Postoperatively topical prednisolone, 1% q.i.d., and a cycloplegic (for example, Cyclogyl 1%), 1 drop at bedtime, are given for 3 or 4 days. No patch is required the day after surgery, and the patient may leave the hospital.

Complications

Complications are few. There is a danger of injury to the ciliary body and hemorrhage if the limbal incision is made too far posteriorly. It may be difficult to prolapse the iris if the pupil is very miotic and especially if the limbal incision is made too far posteriorly. Failure to obtain a watertight closure of the incision can lead to a flat anterior chamber, and immediate surgical repair is mandatory. The other complications listed under peripheral iridectomy with a corneal incision can also occur.

LASER IRIDOTOMY

An alternative to surgical peripheral iridectomy in angle closure glaucoma is iridotomy using the continuous wave form (c-w) argon laser adapted to the slit lamp (Abraham, 1975; Podos et al., 1979; Pollack, 1979). The laser iridotomy is performed as an office procedure in a closed eye—a considerable advantage over surgical iridectomy. It is an effective way of producing an opening in the iris but should not be used in congested or inflamed eyes. Clear media are essential.

Aspirin by mouth (two tablets) and pilocarpine 4% in the affected eye are sometimes used before commencing laser treatment (Podos et al., 1979). The aspirin possibly minimizes prostaglandin reaction and subsequent inflammatory activity in the anterior chamber, whereas the pilocarpine, by placing the iris on stretch, possibly facilitates the procedure. We have not found pilocarpine drops as useful as the literature suggests and do not pretreat patients unless the pupil is 2 mm or more in diameter. The eye is prepared with topical anesthesia. The surgeon should have comfortable arm supports.

Laser Settings

Preliminary stretch burns have been advocated to facilitate the iridotomy. In our experience, creating the stretch burn is generally unnecessary if the Abraham contact lens is used.

A stretch effect is created by a continuous wave argon laser beam of 200-μ spot size with an energy level of 1.0 watt power for 0.1 or 0.2 second; four burns are made into the full thickness iris stroma at each corner of the selected crypt. These burns immediately cause iris contraction and put the crypt on stretch.

Technique

We recommend use of the Abraham lens, which greatly facilitates the procedure. The gonioscopic fluid must be free of air bubbles. The lens is a modified Goldmann fundus lens with a + 66D button and has an antireflective coating. It serves to (1) concentrate the laser energy on the iris; (2) dissipate some of the laser-induced heat from the cornea by defocusing the beam as it passes through the cornea; (3) magnify the area of the iris selected for iridotomy, making it easier to precisely place

the laser burns and to recognize the end point of the procedure, i.e., a through-and-through opening in the iris; (4) stabilize the eye; (5) increase the area of iris exposed by widening the palpebral fissure; and (6) prevent blinking.

An iris crypt one-half to one-third of the distance from the periphery to the pupil in the upper half of the iris is optimal. When the cornea is quite clear, a more peripheral site may be used. An extreme peripheral site should be avoided to prevent endothelial burns. An arcus senilis should also be avoided, as the dense arcus absorbs too much laser energy, thus reducing the chance for a successful iridotomy. The stroma is thinner at an iris crypt, and penetration is facilitated. When no crypt is present, a relatively depigmented area which is slightly thinner than the surrounding stroma can often be found in the mid-periphery. In a blue iris a good site is a suitably placed iris freckle.

We recommend an initial single burn of 500 μ with a 0.5 watt power setting of 0.2 second duration, which often facilitates the procedure. This initial burn is referred to as a "hinge." The spot size is then reduced to 100 μ or 50 μ and energy levels are increased to 0.75 to 1.5 watts for 0.1 to 0.2 second, depending on iris thickness and color. A rapid sequence of burns is made at the center of the iris crypt or the center of the initial burn. The surgeon should aim to use the lowest energy levels that achieve iris penetration. This depends on experience with the technique. An experienced surgeon burning a lightly pigmented iris may produce an iridotomy using 0.5 watt and 0.1 second duration.

Further application of burns should be stopped if (1) no visible response occurs; (2) the corneal epithelium shows burns which manifest as multiple, milky spots on the cornea; (3) endothelial burns (opacities) are seen; (4) the anterior chamber becomes turbid from pigment dispersion; (5) 100 to 150 burns have been applied at one session.

In all these circumstances, a second session is necessary. In most cases (about 80%), an iridotomy is achieved at the first sitting.

As penetration of the iris stroma reaches the pigmented epithelium of the iris, dense bursts of pigment appear in the anterior chamber ("smoke signals"). Power should be reduced by about 50% as the pigment epithelium is easily penetrated. When the pigment epithelium is actually penetrated, a mushroom cloud of aqueous and pigment slowly balloons through the iridotomy site and the anterior chamber deepens. Gonioscopy at this point reveals a more open angle than that noted prior to iridotomy.

At this time, the iridotomy may be enlarged, if it is small. It should be enlarged by treating the pigment epithelium ("chipping away") at the margins of the opening with the same settings, or the spot size may be increased to 100 μ. Loose pigment inside the iridotomy and residual strands of iris stroma running across the center of the iridotomy should be eliminated if possible by laser burning.

Confirmation of a Patent Iridotomy

Patency of the iridotomy is checked at the end of the procedure by noting a red reflex in the iridotomy on retro-illumination and by the visualization of lens capsule on direct slit lamp examination. A considerable amount of pigment may be seen in the anterior chamber at the end of the procedure. This absorbs rapidly and rarely causes any problems.

The patient should be detained in the office for at least 1½ to 3 hours postoperatively to check the intraocular pressure at this time, and a gonioscopy is done to ensure that the angle is open. If the pressure is elevated, appropriate medication is given.

Disadvantage

Laser iridotomy is less likely to be successful during the acute phase of angle closure glaucoma because of corneal edema, ocular congestion and lack of anterior chamber clarity from the turbidity of an inflammatory exudate. The fibrinous exudate that follows laser iridotomy may precipitate a second pressure elevation, resulting in closure of a previously patent iridotomy. Surgical iridectomy is the preferred procedure in cases of acute congestive glaucoma.

Results

The results with laser iridotomy have been encouraging and, in noninflamed eyes, well over 80% of iridotomies are successful. Complications have been few and relatively benign:

1. Localized lens opacities at the site of the iridotomy.

2. Corneal burns which resolve after a few days.

3. Pupil distortion.

4. Transitory iritis with pigment dispersion.

5. Pigment hyperplasia. This may block the iridotomy opening, commonly after 2 to 3 weeks. It requires laser retreatment.

6. Transient rise of intraocular pressure, sometimes to high levels (40 mm Hg or more) a few hours after the procedure. Intraocular pressure should be measured 2 to 3 hours after the procedure.

7. Rare cases have been described of corneal decompensation requiring transplant.

Following laser iridotomy, the patient continues using miotics for at least 3 weeks until permanent patency of the iridotomy is established. Topical steroid drops may be given on the same day and will usually suffice to control postoperative inflammation (prednisolone 1.0% every 2 hours). A cycloplegic is rarely necessary since the iritis is mild and transient and has usually totally resolved by the following morning.

The application of the Yag laser can facilitate the attainment of peripheral iridotomy by utilizing high energy at very short exposures. This is the preferred technique in the light blue iris.

Chapter 8

SURGERY FOR PRIMARY AND SECONDARY OPEN ANGLE AND CHRONIC CLOSED ANGLE GLAUCOMA

FILTERING SURGERY AND LASER TRABECULAR SURGERY

The Filtering Operations: Historical Review (after Sugar, 1981)

Filtering operations for glaucoma date back to the early 19th century. An excellent and comprehensive history of filtering operations has recently been written by Sugar (1981). DeWecker, in 1867 and 1871, introduced the idea of "anterior sclerotomy" in the chamber angle area with an overlying conjunctival bridge flap as a means of producing a filtering cicatrix through which the intraocular fluid might leave the interior of the eye.

In 1894 deWecker added irido-dialysis to the sclerotomy. In many cases the sclerotomy procedures were followed by digital massage and miotics but, in spite of these aids, use of the operation as a primary procedure declined, and it was used by less than 15% of ophthalmologists in the first decade of the 1900's. Successful results a year or more after the operation were few.

Observations of at least temporary successful iridectomy or sclerotomy led to recognition of conjunctival and iris inclusions in the wound. These led to attempts to maintain fistulas through the use of conjunctival infolding into the anterior chamber, iris inclusion and setons.

In 1907, Herbert Herbert introduced his small flap sclerotomy in which a rectangular trap door of sclera was formed with its base attached to the cornea. In 1913 he isolated a wedge of sclera at-tached only to conjunctiva to produce fistulization through shriveling of the isolated wedge. In 1906, Lagrange presented his "sclerecto-iridectomy" which became very popular and has been used to the present time, especially in Europe.

The first iris inclusion sclerectomy operation was introduced in 1857 by George Critchett, as "iridesis." It was defined as the formation of an artificial pupil by tying the iris. The iris was grasped and drawn out of a limbal wound just enough to enlarge the pupil. A silk suture was tied over the prolapsed iris and removed the next day. The development of sympathetic ophthalmia in iris inclusion operations was reported in 1882 by Critchett.

In 1906 Holth, who had the advantage of using the newly available Schiotz tonometer, reported on a procedure he called "iridencleisis antiglaucomatosa." It was based on the premise that effective conjunctival covering over the iris was essential to preserve the integrity of the eye. He made a scleral keratome incision through a sub-Tenon's tunnel with the conjunctival opening some 8 to 10 mm distant from the scleral wound, which was 1 mm from the corneo-limbal junction. The iris sphincter was drawn into the wound and a meridional cut made through it on one side of the forceps. In spite of a high success rate (86%), professional opposition to the operation led Holth to use a modified Lagrange sclerectomy in which a punch instead of scissors was used for the sclerectomy. Later he returned to the iridencleisis operation. An important variation in the iridencleisis operation technique was that introduced by Weekers, who incarcerated two iris tongues into the respective ends of the limbal incision.

The final modification of the early sclerectomy operation came in 1909 when the trephine operation was introduced by Fergus and Elliot.

A large limbus-based triangular scleral flap was made and a 2-mm trephine placed as close to the corneo-limbal junction as possible. Subsequently Elliot modified the procedure by splitting the cornea. The 2-mm trephining was thus half in cornea and half in limbus. An iridectomy was usually made, and the conjunctival flap was repaired. Elliot stressed the importance of removing a complete disc of Descemet's membrane and not involving the trabecular area.

The Elliot operation became the most popular antiglaucoma operation until about 1940, when the relatively high incidence of bleb rupture and late infection led to its decline. Sugar (1950) introduced a trephine operation without splitting the cornea and noted results that showed improvement on previous procedures in older adults with chronic open angle or chronic angle closure glaucoma.

A widely used operation in the 1950's and 1960's was posterior or anterior lip sclerectomy made with a punch forceps and combined with peripheral iridectomy.

TRABECULECTOMY

The first report of a scleral lamellar flap and "experimental trabeculectomy" was by Sugar (1961). The scleral flap was carefully sutured to prevent filtration, but the results were unsuccessful. Cairns subsequently reported very good results, and his basic operation with various modifications is currently the most popular surgical procedure for glaucoma.

In 1958, Scheie introduced a filtering operation using cautery which remained the most popular procedure until the advent of trabeculectomy. Preziosi in 1928 used direct cautery applied obliquely through the sclera to enter the anterior chamber after preparation of a conjunctival flap. The results were very poor.

LASER TRABECULAR SURGERY

Developments in the application of the argon laser to treat angle closure glaucoma led to attempts to use lasers to burn openings through the trabecular meshwork for the treatment of open angle glaucoma (trabeculotomy). These early attempts were unsuccessful (Krasnov, 1973; Worthen and Wickham, 1974; Ticho and Zauberman, 1976).

More recently, Wise and Witter described successful results with open angle glaucoma using low power applications of the argon laser to the trabecular meshwork (Wise and Witter, 1979; Schwartz et al., 1981; Wilensky and Jampol, 1981; Wise, 1981).

We have had good results with this method (Table 8.1). The safety of this mode of treatment when compared to filtering operations makes this a most attractive alternative, and the procedure is rapidly gaining wide acceptance and popularity. A good response and complication-free results are related to the experience and skill of the surgeon. Currently we advise argon laser trabeculoplasty as a first procedure in open angle glaucoma cases which would otherwise require trabeculectomy.

Informed consent should stipulate that there is a small (2 to 3%) risk of sustained increase in intraocular pressure which may necessitate filtration surgery.

TECHNIQUES OF ARGON LASER TRABECULOPLASTY

We have adapted the method described by Wise and Witter, using the argon laser.

The eye is anesthetized with topical anesthetic. A goniolens is applied and the angle visualized. The procedure can be carried out only if the scleral spur is visible. The angle can be best evaluated before commencing the procedure by using the Zeiss four-mirror goniolens and pressing on the cornea to deepen the angle.

The laser is set at $50\text{-}\mu$ aperture size, 0.1 second duration and 0.75 watt power. The laser beam is

Table 8.1 Argon Laser Trabeculoplasty
Results of laser trabeculoplasty in 232 eyes followed for an average of 6 months. Note the average reduction of intraocular pressure by 10.3 mm Hg in phakic eyes and 7.6 mm Hg in aphakic eyes. The intraocular pressure stabilized after 4 to 8 weeks.

	215 Phakic Eyes	17 Aphakic Eyes
Average age	68.4	70.2
Preop intraocular pressure	25.1	25.5
1–7 days	18.8	20.8
2–3 weeks	17.0	21.7
4–8 weeks	15.9	20.2
12–16 weeks	15.8	19.5
20–26+ weeks	14.8	17.8
Average change	−10.3	−7.6
% on fewer medications	20%	5.9%

aimed through a Goldmann three-mirror coated goniolens into the angle anterior to the scleral spur in the anterior trabeculum, ideally at the pigment band situated in the area of the canal of Schlemm (Figs. 8.1 and 8.2). The easiest approach is to divide the angle into four quadrants and start applications at the temporal side of the superior quadrant working around the angle in a counterclockwise direction. Visualization of the angle is enhanced by having the patient look in the direction opposite the quadrant of the angle being treated. Twenty-five burns are applied to each quadrant, spacing them as equally as possibly and applying eight burns for each clock hour. In this way, a total of 100 burns would be applied over 360 degrees. The authors now use 50 burns over 180 degrees applied at each sitting. This is at present the most widely used method because the risk of complications is reduced and the maximum pressure-lowering effect is often achieved with the first session. Otherwise, the remaining 180 degrees of the angle can be treated at another time.

It is important to burn the trabecular meshwork by just the correct amount. The power level is initially set at 0.75 watt and increased if no visible effect on the trabecular meshwork is observed. Further power increases are made until blanching with or without a small gas bubble is observed. This is the ideal power setting. Large gas bubbles must be avoided, and the power should be appropriately reduced if this effect is seen.

In the not uncommon situation where the angle is too narrow to permit adequate visualization of the trabecular meshwork, usually in the superior quadrants, it is often expeditious to combine the technique of gonioplasty (iridoplasty) or tangential photocoagulation of the iris root (or more correctly the last roll of the iris) with standard trabeculoplasty. Gonioplasty is effective in opening the narrow angle as long as no peripheral anterior synechiae have formed. Four to six burns usually suffice for one quadrant. The settings used are 100 to 200 μ, 0.5 watt and 0.1 or 0.2 second duration. The burns cause the iris to shrink away from the cornea

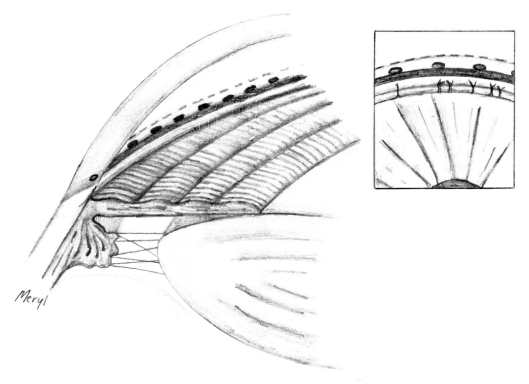

Figure 8.1. Laser trabeculoplasty. Diagrammatic representation of the placement of laser burns for the trabeculoplasty procedures. Laser burns are placed in the anterior trabecular meshwork behind Schwalbe's line and anterior to the pigment line indicating the anatomic location of the canal of Schlemm. Placement of the burns in this area will prevent the formation of peripheral anterior synechiae, which is a major complication if the burns are placed closer to the iris root. For this procedure, an aperture of 0.50 μ is used with 0.1 second duration and 0.50 to 1.0 watt power. Approximately 25 burns are placed in one quadrant, and it is our practice to do two quadrants with 50 burns at one session.

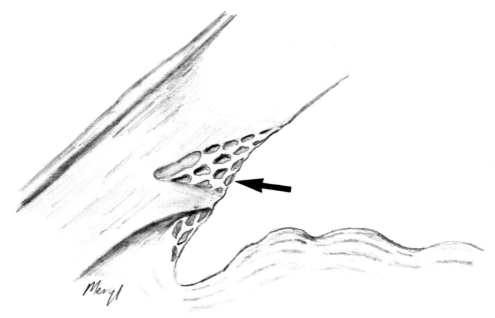

Figure 8.2. Laser trabeculoplasty (continued). This is a diagrammatic representation of the angle of the anterior chamber showing the iris root, ciliary body band, scleral spur and trabecular meshwork with canal of Schlemm anterior to the scleral spur. The *arrow* points to the ideal site, just anterior to the scleral spur, for the laser burns in trabeculoplasty surgery.

and open the angle. This response of the iris enables one to determine adequacy of the settings.

Complications

Postoperatively, a mild inflammatory reaction may require the use of topical steroids, but this is not generally necessary. Complications are rare and usually not significant apart from the rare patient who develops sustained high intraocular pressure. Other complications are iritis, hemorrhage, peripheral anterior synechiae, corneal burns and endothelial decompensation.

LASER IN PSEUDOPHAKIA

Pupil Block

Pupil block in pseudophakos occurs mostly with iris-supported lenses. Argon laser iridotomy is the preferred treatment, using the same technique as described in Chapter 7.

Open Angle Glaucoma with Aphakia and Pseudophakos

Argon laser trabeculoplasty should be attempted using the technique as described above. Care must be taken not to hit the intraocular lens with the laser beam because this may damage the lens. Photocoagulation of ciliary processes through the iridectomy may be useful (Fig. 8.3).

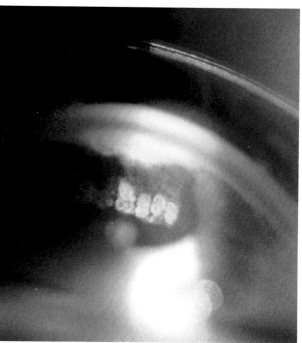

Figure 8.3. Ciliary processes after argon laser photocoagulation. (Courtesy Dr. D. Gorman.)

SURGICAL TECHNIQUES FOR TRABECULECTOMIES, SUBSCLERAL SCHEIE AND CYCLOCRYOTHERAPY

There is no single "trabeculectomy" operation. The technique as originally described by Cairns

(1968) has been so extensively modified that a number of different operations have emerged under the umbrella of "trabeculectomy." These operations can be grouped into three different approaches. The use of an operating microscope is advisable at magnification of 5× to 10×, depending on the stage of the operation.

Keratectomy and Trabeculectomy Extending to the Scleral Spur and Covered by a One-half Thickness or One-third Thickness Scleral Flap Which Is Tightly Sutured to Its Bed

This method has the great advantage of carrying a very low risk of postoperative complications. This advantage is lost in the other two methods. A useful modification of this operation is to use a fornix-based conjunctival flap.

CONJUNCTIVAL FLAP (5× to 7× MAGNIFICATION)

A fornix-based conjunctival flap 7 mm long is raised at the limbus, preferably in the upper nasal quadrant (Fig. 8.4). The conjunctiva and Tenon's fascia are dissected back in a natural surgical plane between themselves and the episclera and sclera (Fig. 8.5). There is minimal dissection of Tenon's fascia compared to a limbus-based flap. Any bleeding points on the flap or episclera are dealt with at this stage.

SCLERAL FLAP (5× TO 7× MAGNIFICATION, #75 BEAVER BLADE WITH 15 DEGREE ANGLE)

The scleral surface is cleaned and a 3 mm × 3 mm scleral flap is outlined with cautery in the exposed sclera. This flap is hinged at the limbus which ensures that the conjunctival and scleral suture lines are separated (Fig. 8.6).

The scleral flap is incised with two one-half thickness radial scleral incisions 3 mm apart, extending back for 3 mm from the limbus (Fig. 8.7). These are joined posteriorly by a 3 mm long incision which is dissected down to the outer surface of the pars plana. The thickness of the sclera can be estimated from the posterior incision allowing accurate dissection of scleral flaps of varying thickness. The thickness chosen for the scleral flap depends on the pathology and the prognosis for surgery. Ideally, the flap should be one-third the scleral thickness, which permits adequate aqueous filtration but avoids the possibility of an excessively thin scleral flap becoming staphylomatous (Fig. 8.8). In patients with a poor prognosis for surgery and in whom better drainage is required, the scleral flap can be dissected thinner than one-third scleral thickness. The dissection of the scleral flap is commenced from the posterior incision at the desired thickness (Fig. 8.8). Staying in the same surgical plane, the flap is carried forward to the cornea to just within the surgical limbus (Fig. 8.9) using a

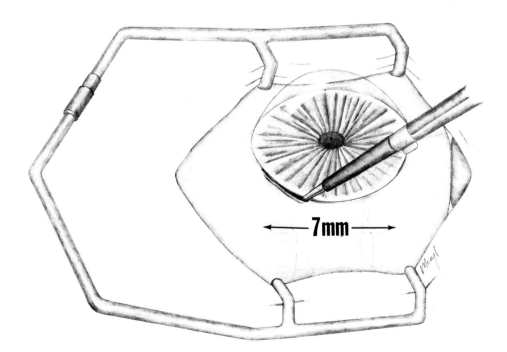

Figure 8.4. Trabeculectomy. A 7 mm long fornix-based conjunctival flap is raised at the limbus using a knife with a microblade (#75 Beaver blade).

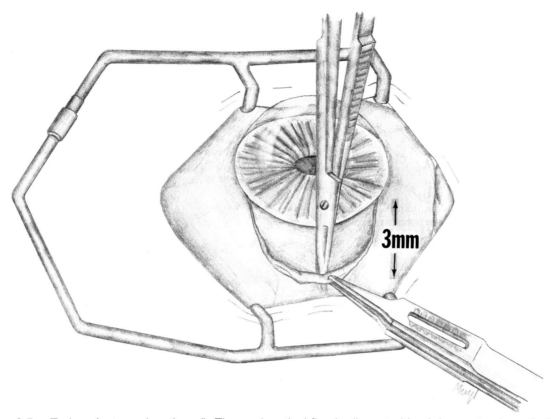

Figure 8.5. Trabeculectomy (continued). The conjunctival flap is dissected back in a natural surgical plane between the conjunctiva, episclera and sclera. At least 3 mm of sclera are exposed between the limbus and the edge of the conjunctival flap.

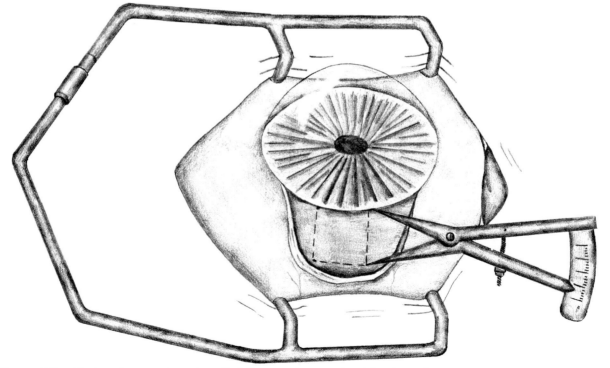

Figure 8.6. Trabeculectomy (continued). A 3 mm × 3 mm scleral flap is outlined with cautery in the exposed sclera.

Figure 8.7. Trabeculectomy (continued). The scleral flap is incised along its radial boundaries to half the depth of the sclera extending back from the limbus for 3 mm using a knife and microblade. In this illustration, a section has been cut through the proximal radial incision into the eye to demonstrate the anatomy underlying the scleral flap that is being fashioned. The scleral flap overlies anteriorly deep lamellae of the cornea. Behind that is the anterior trabeculum extending back to the scleral spur with the canal of Schlemm adjacent to the spur, and extending behind the scleral spur is the posterior trabeculum, the angle of the anterior chamber and the longitudinal and circular muscles of the ciliary body.

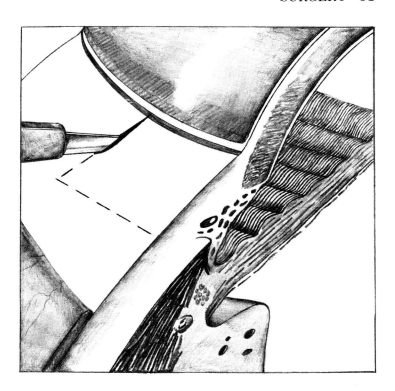

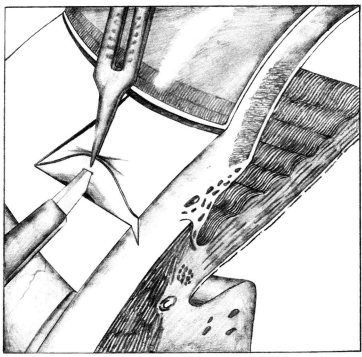

Figure 8.8. Trabeculectomy (continued). The scleral flap has been incised to half the scleral thickness along the radial incisions. The two radial incisions have been joined posteriorly by a 3 mm long incision which is dissected to the surface of the pars plana. By lifting the posterior edge of the flap, the surgeon can visualize the full thickness of the sclera and in this way estimate accurately the thickness of the scleral flap to be dissected. Ideally, the flap should be one-third the scleral thickness. In the illustration the posterior lip of the scleral flap is elevated and a microblade is inserted into the sclera at one-third its depth, starting the dissection of the scleral flap. If more extensive drainage is required, the flap can be made thinner.

hockey stick-shaped disposable Grieshaber blade #68-101 (Beaver blade equivalent #57).

Anatomic Landmarks

With the scleral flap retracted, the salient external landmarks are easily recognized in the deeper undissected tissues (Figs. 8.9 to 8.11). Anteriorly, there is transparent deep corneal tissue; behind this is a gray band of parallel-fibered trabecular tissue which merges posteriorly into white, opaque sclera with crisscrossing fibers. At the junction of the gray trabecular band and the sclera is the scleral spur and Schlemm's canal. This external landmark for the scleral spur and of Schlemm's canal is by far the most important surgical landmark. It indicates the posterior limit of the dissection of corneo-tra-

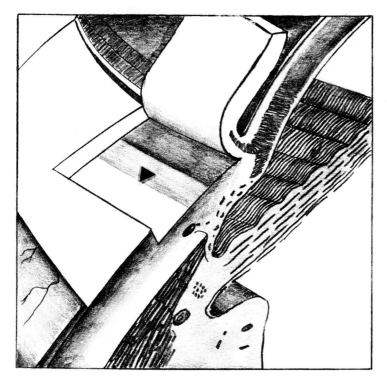

Figure 8.9. Trabeculectomy (continued). The dissection of the scleral flap, shown at its commencement in Figure 8.5, is carried forward in the same surgical plane to just within the surgical limbus. With the flap retracted, the salient external anatomic landmarks are easily visible in the deeper scleral tissues. Anteriorly, the deep cornea lamellae are visible as a transparent band, indicated in the illustration by the *darkly shaded area*. Behind this band is a gray band of parallel-fibered trabecular tissue which merges posteriorly into white, opaque sclera. The junction of the gray trabecular band and the sclera is the scleral spur, and this also indicates the position of Schlemm's canal. In the illustration, it is indicated by an *arrow*. The canal of Schlemm may lie either behind the scleral spur, as shown in this illustration, or overlying the scleral spur or in front of it. The junction of the trabecular meshwork and sclera indicates the posterior limit of dissection in a Cairn's type of trabeculectomy.

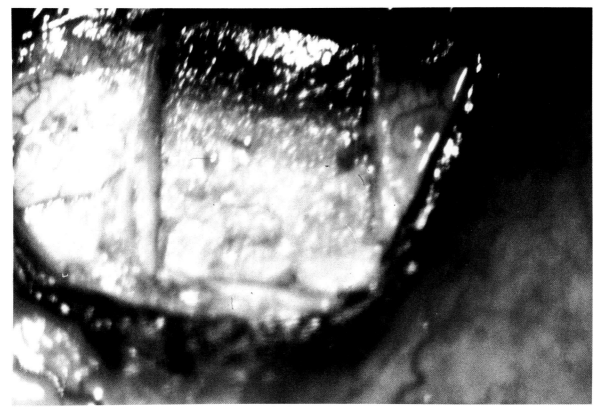

Figure 8.10.

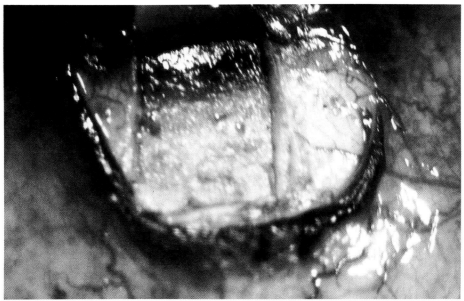

Figure 8.11.

Figures 8.10 and 8.11. Trabeculectomy (continued). These are 35-mm color slides of the surgical procedure taken through the operating microscope. These photographs are taken at the same stage as that indicated in Figure 8.9. The dissection of the superficial one-third thickness of the 3 mm × 3 mm lamellar scleral flap has been completed. The cornea is at the upper part of the slide. The lamellar scleral flap is hinged at the cornea and rotated anteriorly over the cornea, exposing deeper structures. It is just visible in the photograph. In the bed of the dissection, the salient landmarks described in Figure 8.9 are recognized. Anteriorly in the photograph is a transparent band representing corneal lamellae. Posterior to this is a bluish-gray narrower band, which is the trabecular tissue. Behind the trabecular tissue is sclera. The most important landmark is the junction of the posterior border of the trabecular band and the sclera, which represents the external landmark for the scleral spur. The canal of Schlemm has a close relationship to the scleral spur.

becular tissue which is removed in a Cairns' type of trabeculectomy. A pair of preplaced 10-0 nylon sutures is placed from the two posterior corners of the scleral flap to the posterior corners of the flap bed and pulled out of the way (Fig. 8.16).

Using a #75 Beaver blade with a 15 degree angle, the next step is to outline a square 2 mm wide flap in the undissected cornea and trabecular meshwork in the bed of the scleral flap, extending back from the limbus to be hinged at the scleral spur, incising to one-half the depth of this tissue. The anterior incision is made 2 mm long at the base of the initial scleral flap, which at this level is in corneal tissue (Fig. 8.12). Two radial incisions from each end of the anterior incision extend back to the scleral spur (Fig. 8.13) (i.e., junction of the blue trabecular band and sclera). This is approximately 2 mm from the anterior incision, placing it over the scleral spur and canal of Schlemm (Fig. 8.14). With the 2 mm × 2 mm internal flap outlined, the anterior incision is dissected through Descemet's membrane into the anterior chamber. It should be noted that the chamber is not lost at this stage as iris will plug the incision.

10× MAGNIFICATION

The dissection into the anterior chamber is made slowly, using a sharp, pointed microblade with a 15 degree angle (for example, a #75 Beaver blade). Using the knife, the anterior incision at one corner is slowly dissected through Descemet's membrane until the anterior chamber is entered through a small opening, allowing aqueous humor to seep through slowly until the eye becomes soft, but without losing the anterior chamber. In this way, the eye is decompressed slowly. Slow decompression should be practiced in all cases, but particularly in eyes with considerable atrophy of the optic nerve head.

Once the eye has softened, the incision into the anterior chamber is enlarged by careful dissection with the microblade until the opening is large enough to introduce a straight or angled Vannas scissor with which the anterior incision is completed, without losing the anterior chamber. The radial incisions on each side are similarly completed and cut posteriorly to the previously described landmark for the scleral spur (Fig. 8.15). The flap so formed is removed by a posterior incision at the scleral spur which runs parallel to the limbus (Figs. 8.16 and 8.17). The flap of tissue removed consists of cornea, anterior trabecular meshwork and a portion of the scleral spur with or without the canal of Schlemm, depending on its relationship to the scleral spur (Figs. 8.16 and 8.17).

On postoperative gonioscopy, the trabeculectomy opening is seen to extend anteriorly into the cornea, is well anterior to the iris root and extends posteriorly to the scleral spur (Fig. 8.24). The anterior chamber is still maintained, as iris will plug the trabeculectomy opening (Fig. 8.16).

IRIDECTOMY (10× MAGNIFICATION)

An iridectomy is now made. It is imperative that the iridectomy is wider than the trabeculectomy

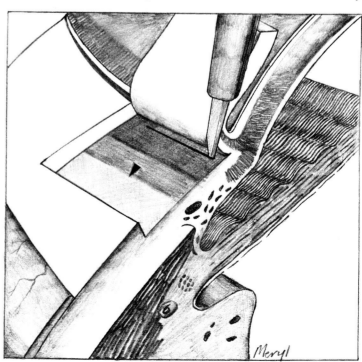

Figure 8.12. Trabeculectomy (continued). An incision is made into cornea extending through approximately one-half thickness of the remaining cornea at the base of the scleral flap. This is the anterior incision for the trabeculectomy.

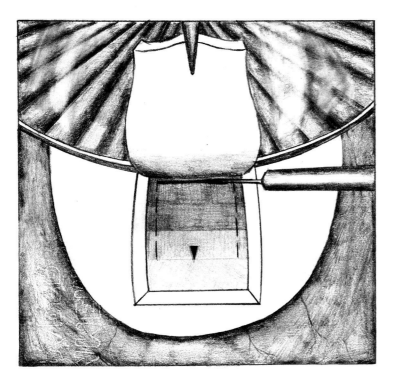

Figure 8.13. Trabeculectomy (continued). This illustration demonstrates the outline of the trabeculectomy flap which is excised. The anterior incision, indicated in the previous illustration, is being completed. This incision is approximately 2 mm in length, thus leaving a small platform on either side. Two radial incisions are made from each end of the anterior incision to the scleral spur extending through half the thickness of the corneal lamellae and the trabecular meshwork. The scleral spur is at the junction of the posterior limit of the trabecular band and sclera and is indicated in the illustration by an *arrow*. These landmarks are easily visible and are indicated in Figures 8.8 and 8.9.

Figure 8.14. Trabeculectomy (continued). The diagram shows a cut through the eye illustrating the anatomy of the area. In the diagram, one sees the anterior trabeculectomy incision in the corneal lamellae extending to half its thickness, and the knife is completing the distal radial incision which has traversed cornea and is in the trabecular band. The trabeculectomy flap is dissected over cornea and anterior trabeculum as far back as the scleral spur. All or part of the canal of Schlemm will be included, depending on its relationship to the scleral spur. With the flap outlined, the anterior incision at the base of the scleral flap is deepened with the microblade until the anterior chamber is entered.

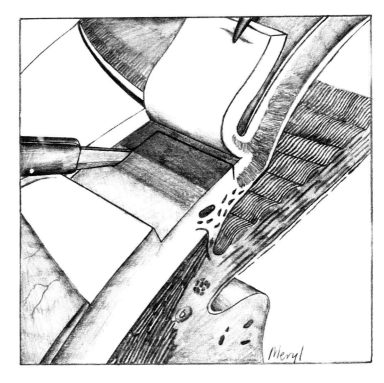

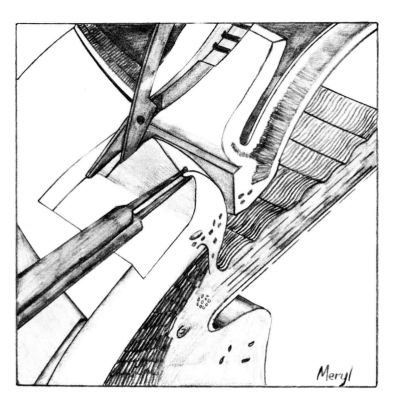

Figure 8.15. Trabeculectomy (continued). The radial incisions for the trabeculectomy are cut with Vannas scissors once the anterior incision has been opened into the anterior chamber. The two radial incisions are cut at full thickness back to the scleral spur, and the flap so formed is hinged on the scleral spur. The opening into the anterior chamber at this point is still plugged by iris, so the anterior chamber is not lost.

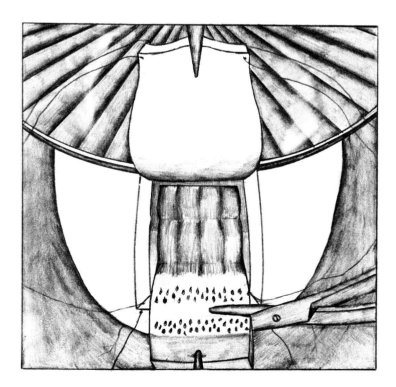

Figure 8.16. Trabeculectomy (continued). The opening made into the anterior chamber is plugged by iris, and the square of tissue that will be removed to complete the trabeculectomy is hinged at the scleral spur. Anteriorly, and hinged at the limbus, is the superficial scleral flap that was originally dissected. Note that two preplaced 10-0 nylon sutures are in position at each of the posterior corners of the scleral flap. The trabeculectomy flap to be excised is shown inferiorly in the illustration, hinged at the scleral spur. One is looking at the anterior chamber side of this flap and can recognize the trabeculectomy opening plugged by iris, the root of the iris inserting into the scleral spur area, the posterior trabecular zone, internal border of the scleral spur, anterior trabecular meshwork and behind that the corneal lamellae which are being held with forceps. The Vannas scissor is completing the trabeculectomy excision with a posterior incision immediately in front of the scleral spur. A 2 mm × 2 mm square of tissue is removed which contains cornea, anterior trabecular meshwork, a portion of the scleral spur and some or all of the canal of Schlemm, depending on its position.

opening to prevent the iris pillars from being pushed into this opening postoperatively. This is achieved by grasping the iris with forceps, moving it to the surgeon's right side and commencing an iridectomy incision with scissors from the left side (Fig. 8.18). As this incision approaches the midway point of the iridectomy, the iris is moved across to the left side and put on stretch and the iridectomy completed (Fig. 8.19). At this stage of the operation the trabeculectomy is completed, extending well into cornea anteriorly and posteriorly to the scleral spur, with an iridectomy which is wider than the trabeculectomy opening (Figs. 8.20 and 8.21).

CLOSURE (5× MAGNIFICATION)

As the iridectomy is completed, the anterior chamber will be lost unless the external lamellar scleral flap is quickly repositioned by tying the preplaced 10-0 nylon sutures at the posterior edges of the scleral flap (Fig. 8.21). Balanced salt solution is injected into the anterior chamber to deepen it. The partial thickness scleral flap is securely sutured using four additional interrupted 10-0 nylon sutures. One pair of sutures is placed at each side of the flap at the limbus. These are crucial sutures

and effectively prevent excessive drainage of fluid through the limbal area which could cause leakage through a fornix-based conjunctival flap in the early postoperative phase. The second pair of sutures is placed midway along the flap on each side, and the third pair of sutures are those already tied at the posterior corners of the flap (Fig. 8.22). The scleral flap controls filtration of aqueous from the anterior chamber and prevents postoperative staphyloma formation. The conjunctiva is rotated anteriorly to the limbus and sutured to the episclera and sclera with two 10-0 nylon sutures at each end of the conjunctival flap, pulling the conjunctival edge taut but not tight across the limbus (Fig. 8.23).

Balanced salt solution is injected under the conjunctival flap to lift it from the sclera. The patient leaves the operating table with an intact anterior chamber and a bleb at the site of the trabeculectomy.

ADVANTAGES

The advantages of this technique over the limbus-based flap trabeculectomy are as follows:

1. There is better exposure and visualization of

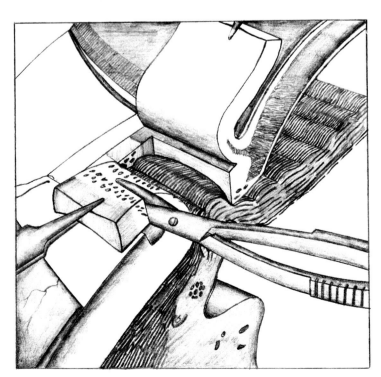

Figure 8.17. Trabeculectomy (continued). Completion of the trabeculectomy excision is achieved with Vannas scissors, making an incision immediately in front of the scleral spur and behind the anterior trabeculum. There is a side cut into the anterior chamber demonstrating the anatomy of the area. The opening is plugged with iris, and at the far side of the trabeculectomy excision one can recognize the cut portion of the cornea and anterior trabecular meshwork in the wall of the radial incision.

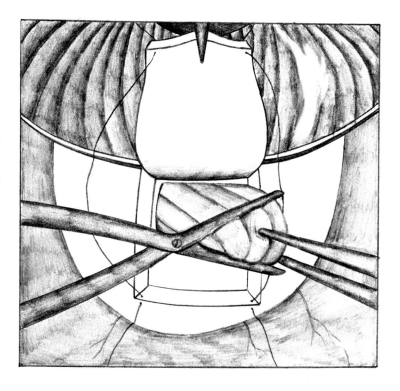

Figure 8.18. Trabeculectomy (continued). Performing the iridectomy is illustrated in this figure and the subsequent figure. The iris is grasped at its center with a pair of Hoskin forceps (#19 or 28) and pulled to the right side. A Vannas scissor is used, cutting from the left halfway through the roll of iris.

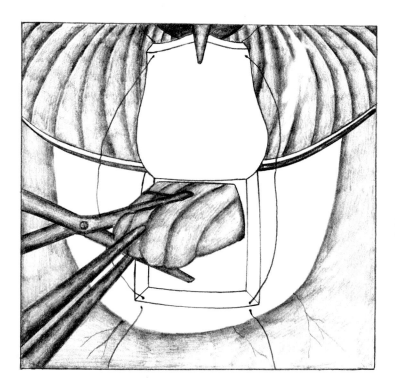

Figure 8.19. Trabeculectomy (continued). The iridectomy is completed by moving the roll of iris to the left side and completing incision of the iris, still cutting with the scissor from the left side.

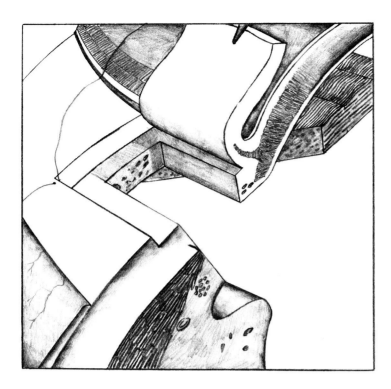

Figure 8.20. Trabeculectomy (continued). The completed trabeculectomy opening showing the iridectomy, which is wider than the trabeculectomy opening.

Figure 8.21. Trabeculectomy (continued). The lamellar scleral flap has been repositioned, and the preplaced 10-0 nylon sutures at the posterior edge of the scleral flap have been tied.

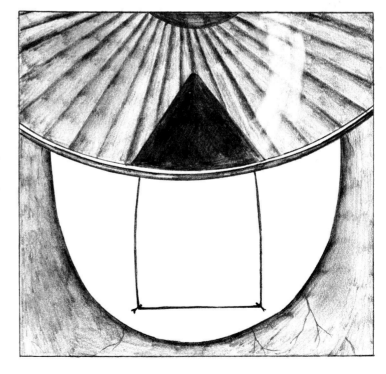

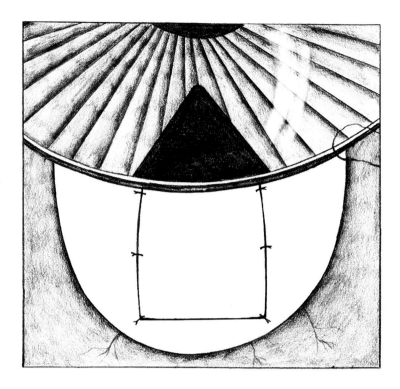

Figure 8.22. Trabeculectomy (continued). The scleral flap is sutured back to the scleral bed with six 10-0 nylon sutures, thus ensuring good closure of the trabeculectomy opening.

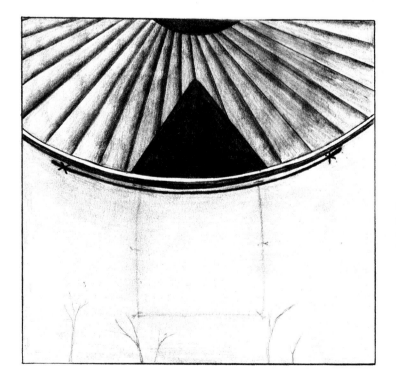

Figure 8.23. Trabeculectomy (continued). The conjunctival closure. The free edge of the conjunctiva is rotated anteriorly to the limbus and sutured with two 10-0 nylon sutures placed through the episclera-sclera and conjunctival edge at each end of the conjunctival flap. The conjunctival edge should fit snugly across the limbus.

the operating field. Dissection of the scleral flap well into the cornea is facilitated (Fig. 8.9). This ensures a trabeculectomy in front of the root of the iris and ciliary body and reduces the possibility of hypertrophic ciliary body pigment or iris adhesions obstructing the trabeculectomy opening (Fig. 8.24).

2. The procedure is technically easier than dissecting a limbus-based flap, especially when operating in an area of conjunctiva scarred from either previous trauma or surgery.

3. The possibility of damaging the conjunctival flap during dissection, especially button-holing the flap, is eliminated.

4. The conjunctival flap adheres and scars at the limbus. The subconjunctival bleb that results is pushed posteriorly, producing a diffuse, well vascularized thicker walled bleb extending toward the upper fornix and not overlying the limbus (Fig. 8.25). There is little possibility of developing a thin, avascular bleb overhanging the cornea.

5. Soft or hard contact lenses can be fitted within

2 weeks after surgery and will not interfere with bleb function.

6. The scleral flap is sutured back into place. The flap prevents excessive aqueous humor filtration and maintains the anterior chamber postoperatively. The rate of aqueous filtration can be varied by altering the thickness of the scleral flap, e.g., a thicker flap will reduce the rate of aqueous filtration.

In advanced refractory glaucoma, the properly sutured scleral flap will diminish the risk of a scleral staphyloma if the intraocular pressure remains high postoperatively.

There is no difference in the average pressure-lowering effect of trabeculectomy when using either a sutured or unsutured flap (Freedman et al., 1976).

7. The same technique with all its advantages can be effectively used for combined cataract surgery and trabeculectomy. The risk of shallow or absent anterior chamber postoperatively is considerably reduced by this method (see Chapter 9).

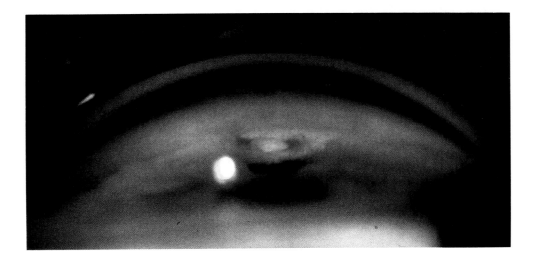

Figure 8.24. Trabeculectomy (continued). A gonioscopic view of the completed trabeculectomy procedure which shows the trabeculectomy in clear cornea well in front of the root of the iris and the ciliary body band and extending posteriorly to the scleral spur. The corneal placement of the trabeculectomy reduces any possibility of hypertrophic ciliary body pigment or iris adhesions obstructing the trabeculectomy opening.

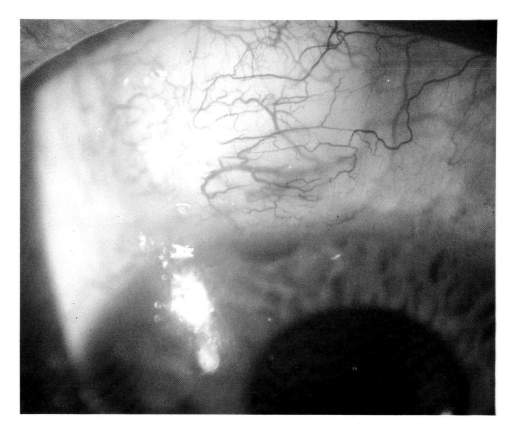

Figure 8.25. Trabeculectomy (continued). The bleb associated with this type of trabeculectomy procedure is a diffuse, well vascularized thick-walled bleb which is usually associated with excellent drainage.

Trabeculectomy and Keratectomy Extending to the Scleral Spur Using a Limbus-based Flap with the Scleral Flap Remaining Unsutured or Loosely Sutured

CONJUNCTIVAL FLAP (5× to 7× MAGNIFICATION)

A 15 mm long conjunctival flap is made with Westcott scissors starting 10 mm from the limbus (Fig. 8.26). Tenon's fascia is included in the flap. The superior rectus muscle tendon is carefully avoided. The flap incision arches in semicircular shape to within 4 mm of the limbus at its extremities. A #64 Beaver blade or similar knife is used to scrape Tenon's fascia at the limbal area into the base of the flap (Fig. 8.27). Episcleral vascular tissue is scraped away from the limbus with a Bard-Parker #15 blade over a wide area. Hemostasis is meticulously obtained using wet field cautery or a disposable cautery lightly applied to the sclera (Fig. 8.28). It is important to avoid deep burns in the sclera which would then produce a "Swiss cheese" appearance when the lamellar dissection is performed.

TRABECULECTOMY (7× to 10× MAGNIFICATION)

A 5 mm square lamellar scleral flap (Fig. 8.29) is cut at approximately one-half to one-third thickness, using a diamond knife or Bard-Parker #15 blade or razor knife (Fig. 8.30). (Our preference is the diamond knife.) The lamellar flap is dissected off its scleral bed, and the dissection is carried into deep cornea for 0.5 mm (Fig. 8.31). Two radial incisions 0.5 mm within the boundaries of the trap door bed are made with the diamond knife or a razor knife, entering the anterior chamber (Fig. 8.32). The cut edges of trabecular meshwork are grasped with Bonn forceps, and both radial incisions are united anteriorly with straight Vannas scissors (Fig. 8.33). The block of deep cornea and trabecular meshwork is held upward. The radial incisions are extended and united posteriorly using Vannas scissors, immediately anterior to a narrow band of ciliary body (usually approximately 0.5 mm width). Iris usually protrudes when the anterior chamber is entered with the Vannas scissors. A small iridotomy made with the scissors allows

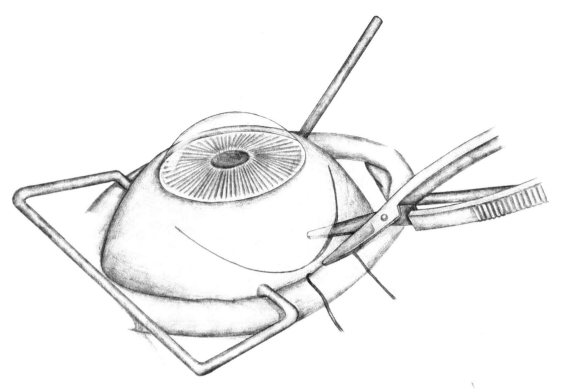

Figure 8.26. Trabeculectomy (continued). A 15 mm long limbus-based conjunctival flap is made with Westcot scissors starting 10 mm from the limbus. Tenon's fascia is included in the flap. The superior rectus muscle tendon is carefully avoided. The conjunctival flap arches in semicircular shape to within 4 mm of the limbus at its extremities.

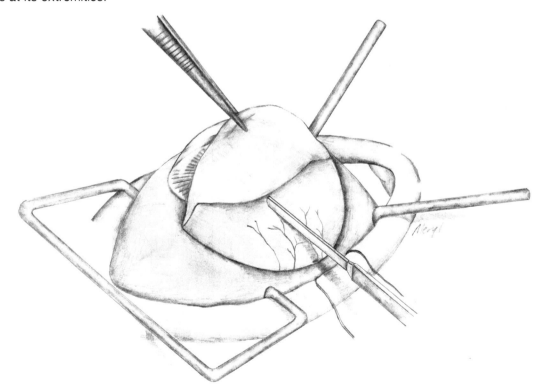

Figure 8.27. Trabeculectomy (continued). A #64 Beaver blade (or Tooke knife) is used to scrape Tenon's fascia at the limbal area into the base of the conjunctival flap. This dissection is carried to just within the surgical limbus.

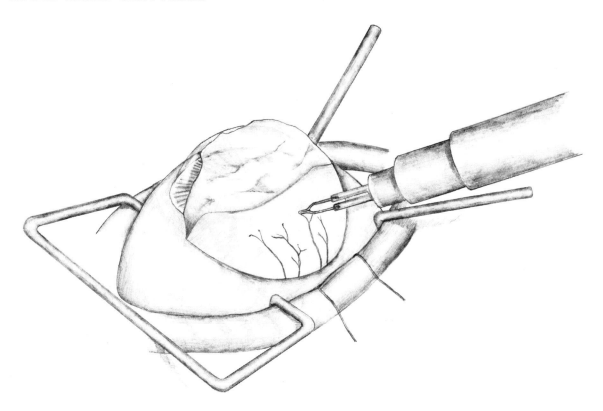

Figure 8.28. Trabeculectomy (continued). Hemostasis is obtained meticulously using disposable cautery or bipolar cautery lightly applied to the sclera. It is important to avoid burning deeply in the sclera, which, if perforated, may result in a "Swiss cheese" appearance in the lamellar dissection.

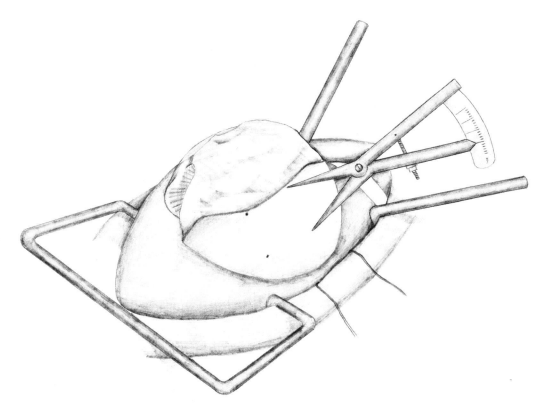

Figure 8.29. Trabeculectomy (continued). A 5 mm square lamellar scleral flap is marked out.

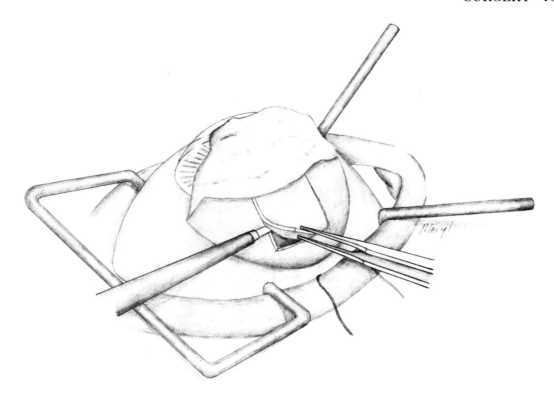

Figure 8.30. Trabeculectomy (continued). The 5 mm square lamellar scleral flap is dissected out using a diamond knife or Bard-Parker #5 blade or razor knife, preferably the diamond knife. The lamellar flap is dissected off its scleral bed starting at the posterior corners.

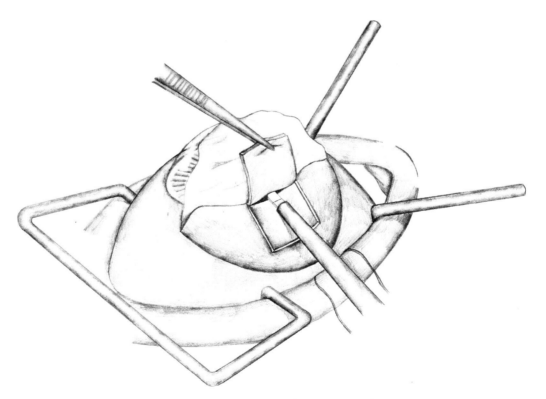

Figure 8.31. Trabeculectomy (continued). Dissection of the lamellar flap is carried anterior to the surgical limbus into deep corneal lamellae for 0.5 mm.

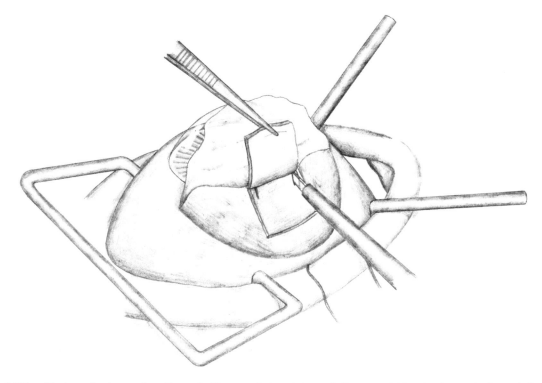

Figure 8.32. Trabeculectomy (continued). Two radial incisions 0.5 mm within the boundaries of the trap door bed are made with a diamond knife or razor knife entering the anterior chamber.

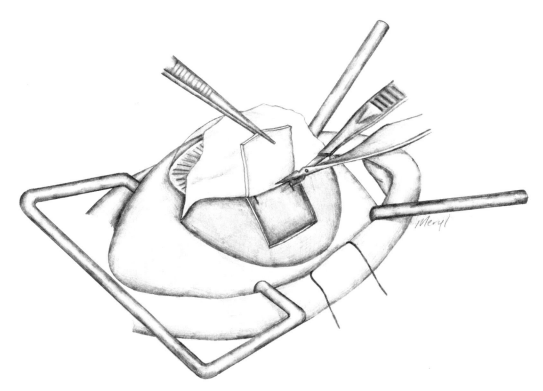

Figure 8.33. Trabeculectomy (continued). The two radial incisions are united anteriorly with straight Vannas scissors, one blade of which is in the anterior chamber.

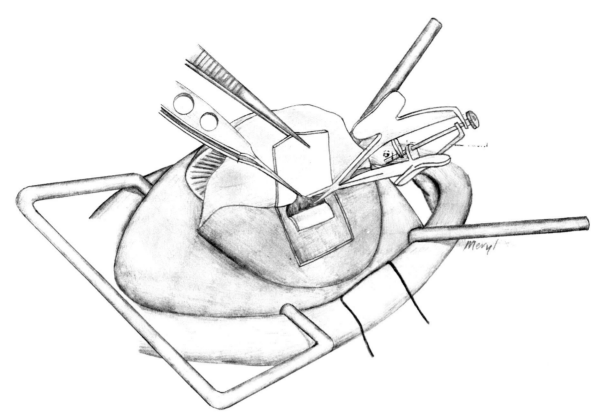

Figure 8.34. Trabeculectomy (continued). Iris usually protrudes when the anterior chamber is entered with the Vannas scissors. A small iridotomy is made, allowing aqueous to escape from the posterior chamber, and the iris falls backward.

aqueous to escape from the posterior chamber and the iris falls back (Figs. 8.34 and 8.35). A wide-based peripheral iridectomy is performed with deWecker scissors exposing several ciliary processes. Hemostasis is completely secured using the bipolar wet field cautery.

CLOSURE (5× MAGNIFICATION)

The scleral flap is repaired with 10-0 nylon sutures at each corner (Fig. 8.36) and optional additional lateral sutures if the anterior chamber is emptied. When bulk flow is desired, e.g., in reoperations, scleral cautery applied to the posterior lip of the scleral flap may encourage distal free egress of aqueous. The conjunctival flap, including Tenon's fascia, is repaired with a continuous 6-0 plain catgut suture (Fig. 8.36). Solumedrol 0.5 cc is injected subconjunctivally in the inferior fornix if severe postoperative reaction is anticipated. One drop of Hyoscine 0.25% is instilled after irrigating the eye with Neosporin or chloramphenicol solution.

COMPLICATIONS

The operation is essentially a "guarded" sclerectomy and does not provide as good a scleral barrier to free filtration as does the tightly sutured scleral flap. If the scleral flap is not sutured at all, the operation carries the same risk of major complications as do the classical full thickness filtering operations—that is, shallow or flat anterior chamber, postoperative hypotony and its sequelae, cataract, malignant glaucoma and the formation of a staphyloma at the site of the operation. A rare but serious complication is sympathetic ophthalmia.

In view of the high risk of complications if the lamellar scleral flap is not sutured, probably without any added intraocular pressure reduction, the surgeon should consider the alternative of using the subscleral Scheie operation when faced with the need to control very high intraocular pressure. This carries the higher risk of complications but has the "benefit" of a greater average reduction of the intraocular pressure. The technique for the subscleral Scheie operation is described below.

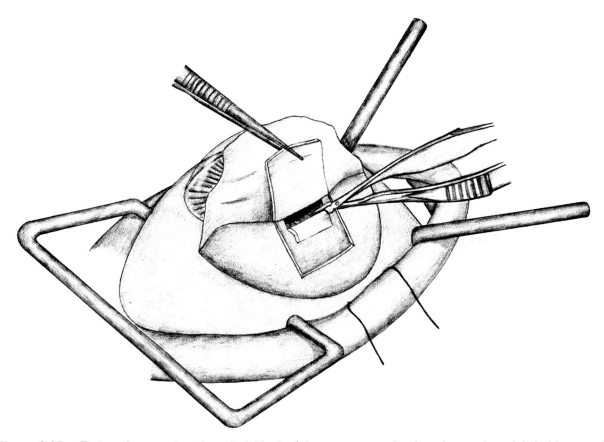

Figure 8.35. Trabeculectomy (continued). A block of deep cornea and trabecular meshwork is held upward, the radial incisions are extended to the scleral spur and the block of tissue is removed with Vannas scissors by a posterior incision.

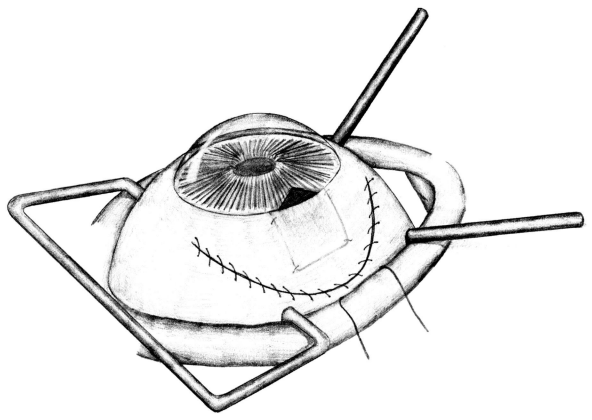

Figure 8.36. Trabeculectomy (continued). The scleral flap is repaired with 10-0 nylon sutures at each posterior corner, and optional additional lateral sutures are added. The conjunctival flap, including Tenon's capsule, is repaired with a continuous 6-0 plain catgut suture.

The "Watson" Trabeculectomy

The operation is a combined keratectomy, sclerectomy and internal cyclodialysis performed under a scleral flap.

CONJUNCTIVAL FLAP (5× MAGNIFICATION)

A fornix-based or limbus-based conjunctival flap is raised, in the same way as described in the previous two operations (Fig. 8.37).

SCLERAL FLAP (7× to 10× MAGNIFICATION)

The scleral surface is cleaned and a one-half thickness 3 mm × 3 mm scleral flap, hinged at the limbus, is dissected and reflected anteriorly over the cornea to expose the deeper scleral layers. Watson described a 4 mm square scleral flap.

The landmarks as previously described are easily recognized—that is, deep corneal tissue anteriorly, behind that a gray band of trabeculum, the junction of its posterior border and the sclera being the

external landmark for the scleral spur, and behind that scleral tissue (Fig. 8.37).

SCLERECTOMY, CYCLODIALYSIS, TRABECULECTOMY (7× to 10× MAGNIFICATION)

Using a #75 Beaver micropoint blade, an incision is made in the deep scleral tissue just anterior to the posterior incision for the scleral flap and parallel to the limbus. This incision is 3 mm wide, and the dissection is carried through sclera into the suprachoroidal space, exposing pars plana (Fig. 8.37). Starting at each end of this incision, two radial incisions are cut approximately 2 mm apart, running anteriorly toward the limbus, using Vannas scissors. These radial incisions are carried forward until the ciliary body attachment to the deep scleral tissue is reached (Fig. 8.38).

A cyclodialysis spatula is introduced under the sclera into the suprachoroidal space, and the attachment of the ciliary body to sclera is separated off by blunt dissection with entry into the anterior chamber (Fig. 8.38). The radial incisions of the

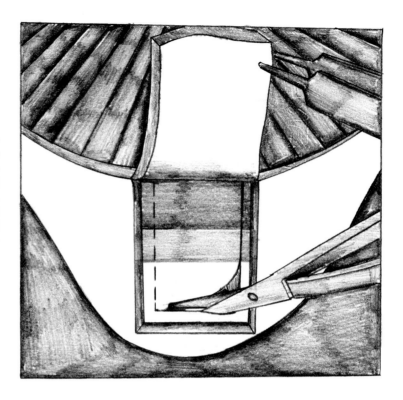

Figure 8.37. Trabeculectomy (continued). "Watson" trabeculectomy. A deep scleral flap is dissected, placing the posterior incision approximately 3 mm behind the limbus dissected to the pars plana. From this posterior incision, using Vannas scissors two radial incisions 2 mm apart are cut running anteriorly toward the limbus.

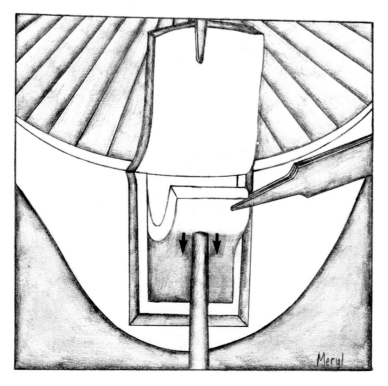

Figure 8.38. Trabeculectomy (continued). The two radial incisions are carried forward until the ciliary body attachment to the scleral spur is reached. A cyclodialysis spatula is introduced under the sclera into the suprachoroidal space to detach ciliary body from the scleral spur by blunt dissection.

deep scleral flap are continued to the limbus as far as the reflection of the superficial scleral flap. The dissection of the 2 mm wide × 3 mm long deep corneo-trabecular-scleral flap is completed with Vannas scissors by an incision joining the two radial incisions anteriorly at the limbus. Removal of the deep scleral flap exposes a 2 mm wide × 3 mm long corneo-scleral opening which extends from the limbus to the scleral spur and for 1 mm behind the scleral spur. An iridectomy is performed.

CLOSURE (5× MAGNIFICATION)

The superficial scleral flap is then rotated back onto its bed to which it is sutured with six interrupted 10-0 nylon sutures, one pair at the limbus, one pair at the posterior corners and one pair midway between these two. The conjunctival flap is then replaced and sutured, the choice of suture depending on the type of flap (limbus-based or fornix-based).

The operation is essentially a combined keratectomy, trabeculectomy and internal cyclodialysis. It is associated with a higher incidence of postoperative complications, particularly uveal effusion and uveitis, and the few documented studies suggest that the surgical result is no better than the results of a trabeculectomy anterior to the scleral spur.

Results of Subscleral Trabeculectomy

With proper selection of cases, the surgeon can expect success in terms of reduction of intraocular pressure (to less than 21 mm Hg) in over 90% of cases. Depending on the technique used, the length of follow-up and the type of glaucoma, approximately 30% to 50% of eyes will require postoperative medication.

Long Term Management

Digital pressure may be valuable starting at approximately 3 to 4 weeks postoperatively when the pressure often goes up from levels below 10 mm Hg to over 20 mm Hg. Excessive massage can cause blockage of the trabeculectomy site with an updrawn pupil, resulting in an acute elevation in the intraocular pressure which reverses spontaneously. Another complication of massage is rupture of Descemet's membrane and acute corneal opacification. A third complication is a mild uveitis. By tapering of topical steroids and stopping the cycloplegics, one can curb the rising pressure and allow better filtration. Visual acuity is checked at each visit by refraction and pin-hole. Maximal visual acuity is usually achieved 3 to 8 weeks postoperatively.

Complications of the Operation

The complications are similar to those of other filtering procedures and are described in Chapter 12. Suturing the scleral flap to its bed reduces the risk of postoperative complications, and it is for this reason that trabeculectomy has become such a popular operation for glaucoma.

With a well sutured scleral flap, the incidence of serious postoperative complications is less than 1% (Luntz, 1980).

TRABECULECTOMY—MODIFICATIONS

Lamellar Scleral Flap

SHAPE

The lamellar scleral flap may be shaped as a limbus-based triangle instead of a square (Fig. 8.39). There is no real advantage in such a triangular flap.

POSITION

The scleral flap may be hinged at the scleral spur rather than the limbus. In this case, the radial incisions are joined by an anterior cut at the limbus which will lie over the trabeculectomy opening and so communicate directly with the anterior chamber. The main disadvantage is the danger of a full thickness fistula developing at the anterior end of the flap, even if it is sutured at the limbus, thus losing its "barrier effect" against excessive filtration.

Trabeculectomy Excision

SHAPE

Incising a triangular rather than a square deep scleral flap, with the base at the limbus or the scleral spur, has no specific advantages.

Round (Trephino-Trabeculectomy, Trepano-Trabeculectomy)

Using a 1½-mm or 2-mm Elliot trephine, a round disc of corneo-trabeculum is removed, leaving a trephine hole (Fig. 8.40). There is danger of damaging the lens when the trephine enters the anterior chamber, particularly if the anterior chamber is shallow. The trephine disc can fall into the anterior chamber, as there is no way of holding it during the trephine cut. No definite advantages for this method have been demonstrated.

TRABECULAR BLOCK USED AS A SETON

There are modifications where the trabecular block is not excised but rotated into the anterior chamber to act as a seton. There are no specific advantages to this method.

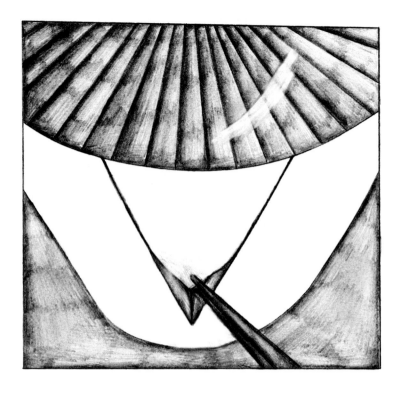

Figure 8.39. Trabeculectomy (continued). Trabeculectomy may be performed using a triangular superficial scleral flap rather than a square.

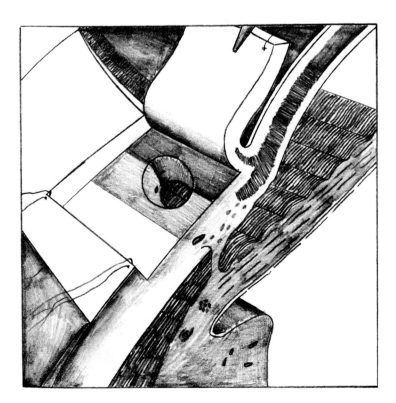

Figure 8.40. Trabeculectomy (continued). A trephine hole straddling the cornea-trabeculectomy junction can be made instead of dissecting out a square trabeculectomy opening. The disadvantage of the trephine is that it is performed "blind."

SUBSCLERAL THERMOSCLERECTOMY (TRABECULECTOMY)

The subscleral thermosclerectomy is a modification of trabeculectomy (as described on pp. 72–79). The wet field cautery is applied to the margins of the window produced by removal of the block of trabecular meshwork and to the distal margin of the lamellar scleral flap which is anchored by sutures only at the corners. Cauterization enlarges the fistula and facilitates subscleral filtration.

HISTOLOGY

Histologic material from trabeculectomy will show cornea and trabeculum (Fig. 8.41) and in a "Watson" trabeculectomy, sclera and ciliary body pigment adherent to the scleral spur (Fig. 8.30).

The canal of Schlemm is usually seen in a specimen from a "Watson" trabeculectomy (Fig. 8.42). but is included in only about 50% of specimens from a trabeculectomy anterior to the scleral spur. This is due to the variable anatomic localization of the canal of Schlemm just anterior to, overlying or immediately behind the scleral spur. If the canal is situated behind the scleral spur, it will not be found in the histologic specimen.

Mode of Action

Trabeculectomy is most probably a filtering operation, because its adequate functioning depends on the formation of a bleb. The way in which aqueous humor filters to the subconjunctival space is not fully understood, but there are four possible mechanisms:

1. Drainage through the cut ends of the canal of Schlemm. These have been shown by histology and electron microscopy to close off by fibrosis after surgery; therefore, this cannot be the way the trabeculectomy operation functions.

2. Drainage through unsutured radial and posterior incisions of the lamellar scleral flap which are presumed to remain open following surgery. A similar drop of intraocular pressure, however, is achieved when the flap is sutured, so this cannot be the major route for filtration.

3. Cairns has suggested that filtration occurs through the cut ends of the collector channels on the deep surface of the lamellar scleral flap. This is

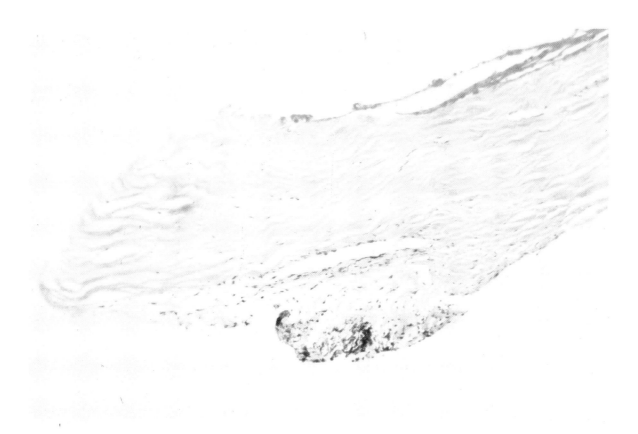

Figure 8.41. Trabeculectomy (continued). Histologic section from a trabeculectomy specimen (Cairns' type) showing cornea, trabeculum and Schlemm's canal.

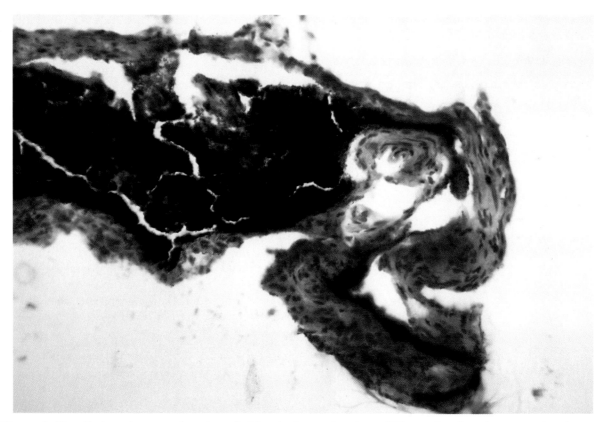

Figure 8.42. Trabeculectomy (continued). Histologic section from "Watson" trabeculectomy showing cornea, trabeculum, canal of Schlemm, sclera and ciliary body pigment adherent to the scleral spur.

one possibility that has not been fully investigated, although the likelihood would be that these cut ends close by fibrosis in the same way as the cut ends of the canal of Schlemm.

4. Another explanation is that there is seepage of aqueous through lamellar sclera which is known to be permeable to aqueous. This can be verified in the laboratory by taking a 1-mm lamellar disc of sclera, fixed in a container and exposed to 21 mm Hg pressure with a vacuum pump. On the other side of the scleral button is a reservoir filled with a colored fluid in contact with the scleral button. Twenty-four hours later the same colored fluid will collect on the reverse side of the scleral button by seeping through the button. The amount of fluid that seeps across the scleral button in unit volume and unit time corresponds closely to the known flow of aqueous in a normal eye (M. H. Luntz, unpublished data).

SUBSCLERAL SCHEIE (SUBSCLERAL THERMOSCLEROSTOMY)

The subscleral Scheie operation or a subscleral thermosclerectomy is preferable to trabeculectomy for secondary glaucoma, chronic angle closure glaucoma and primary open angle glaucoma with high intraocular pressure (greater than 40 mm Hg) (see Chapter 6).

A suitable area of conjunctiva is selected. The best site is virgin, untraumatized conjunctiva and preferably the upper nasal quadrant. Where conjunctival scarring is present, an area of normal or near-normal conjunctiva is selected.

CONJUNCTIVAL FLAP (5× MAGNIFICATION)

Using Westcott scissors, a conjunctival incision 9 mm in length is made in the fornix, 7 mm behind and parallel to the surgical limbus. The incision is carried through the subconjunctival tissue to sclera, and the scleral surface is laid bare. Dissection is then carried forward, using either a Westcott or Troutman scissors, toward the surgical limbus, separating conjunctiva and Tenon's fascia from sclera. Dissection becomes difficult as the limbus is approached where Tenon's capsule and episcleral tissue fuse: a disposable Beaver knife (#75 or #64) is used to dissect into the limbal area. The limbus-based conjunctival flap is rotated forward onto the cornea and held there by an assistant, using a #28 Pierse forceps (Fig. 8.43).

SCLERAL FLAP: (7× to 10× MAGNIFICATION)

A scleral flap hinged at the limbus, extending back 1.0 mm from the limbus and 5 mm in length, is marked out on the sclera beneath the conjunctival flap, using the bipolar cautery. Two radial incisions and a posterior incision are made extending to half the scleral thickness (Fig. 8.44) using a diamond blade, and this one-half thickness scleral flap hinged at the limbus is rotated forward onto the cornea.

FISTULA AND IRIDECTOMY (10× MAGNIFICATION)

Using the diamond knife, a 4 to 5 mm. long incision is made parallel to the limbus into the deep scleral tissue at the base of the anteriorly rotated scleral flap (Fig. 8.45). This incision is carried to half the thickness of the remaining sclera, and a row of cautery burns, preferably using a bipolar cautery, is applied to the posterior wall of the incision (Fig. 8.46). The incision is deepened to Descemet's membrane, and a second row of cautery application is made along the posterior lip beneath the first row. The next step is to enter the anterior chamber using the Beaver knife across the full 4 to 5 mm length of the incision. To do this safely, the surgeon lifts the anterior lip of the incision with a #19 Pierse forceps and the assistant lifts the posterior lip of the incision with a second pair of forceps. Using the Beaver blade, the anterior chamber is entered at one end of the 5 mm long scleral incision, and, with the blade held pointing upward, the incision is carried across to the other end, thus completing the opening into the anterior chamber. Using pressure on the posterior lip of the scleral incision, iris is prolapsed into the incision (Fig. 8.47). If it does not prolapse it should be carefully grasped through the fistula. Grasping the iris with a #28 Hoskin forceps, a peripheral iridectomy is made (Fig. 8.48). The iris is allowed to slip back into the anterior chamber, ensuring that it is not incarcerated in the incision. When this happens, the iris can be freed by using a jet of balanced salt solution through the incision.

CLOSURE (5× MAGNIFICATION)

The conjunctival flap is rotated back into the fornix covering the one-half thickness scleral flap, which is not sutured. Tenon's capsule is sutured with interrupted 10-0 nylon sutures, and an interrupted or continuous 8-0 Vicryl suture unites the cut conjunctival edges (Fig. 8.49). A drop of an antibiotic-steroid combination is instilled into the conjunctival sac at the completion of the surgery.

The scleral flap has two functions:

1. It strengthens the conjunctiva at the limbus. The conjunctiva there is under the greatest pressure from fluid draining through the fistula and often becomes thin, overhangs the cornea and may perforate. The scleral flap prevents this.

2. It acts as a flap directing the flow of aqueous away from the limbus to the posterior portion of the bleb, thereby producing a more diffuse, posterior bleb.

POSTOPERATIVE MANAGEMENT

Fistulizing Operations

A steroid antibiotic combination is useful for a few days postoperatively, depending on the extent of postoperative iritis. As soon as the anterior chamber reaction has improved to a level of 1+ cells and flare, the patient should be weaned off the medication. A mydriatic may be used routinely for 3 to 7 days, or only if the anterior chamber reaction exceeds 1+ cell and flare. This is usually not necessary after fistulizing operations and is very seldom necessary after peripheral iridectomy.

The treatment of complications is described in Chapter 12.

A transient ocular hypertension may follow some fistulizing procedures, particularly trabeculectomy, lasting from 2 days to 6 weeks. The reason for this is obscure, but it may be related to postsurgical edema of the trabeculum, to obstruction of the fistula by blood, to early failure of the bleb or to use of steroids or cycloplegics. If blood is the causative factor, the pressure will gradually drop to a normal postoperative level once the blood has resorbed. Massage used three or four times a day may be helpful during the ocular hypertensive period, each episode of massage lasting 3 to 5 minutes. Some surgeons institute massage routinely as soon as the anterior chamber is reformed, usually the day after surgery, in the belief that this will facilitate bleb formation. We prefer to avoid the use of massage if the patient is doing well, as massage can induce an inflammatory anterior chamber exudate (cells and flare) which may compromise normal bleb formation. Massage should be used only if drainage through the scleral fistula appears to be inadequate.

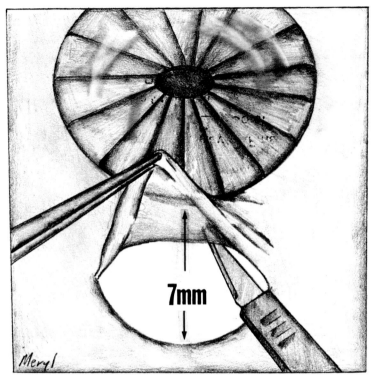

Figure 8.43. A subscleral Scheie operation showing the limbus-based conjunctival flap which has been rotated forward onto the cornea.

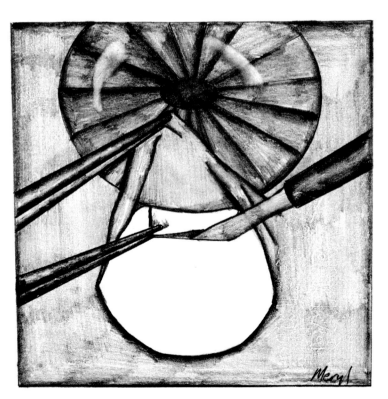

Figure 8.44. Subscleral Scheie (continued). A scleral flap 1.0 mm wide and 5 mm long hinged at the limbus is outlined, and a 5 mm long posterior incision is made extending to half the scleral thickness in depth.

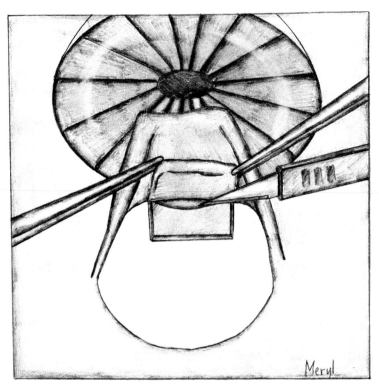

Figure 8.45.   Subscleral Scheie (continued). A scleral flap, 1.0 mm wide and 5 mm long, hinged at the limbus and extending to half the scleral thickness has been dissected and rotated anteriorly onto the cornea resting on the conjunctival flap. A 4.5 mm long incision is made in the scleral bed at the base of the lamellar scleral flap. This incision will become the Scheie fistula.

Figure 8.46.   Subscleral Scheie (continued). Before penetrating the anterior chamber, two rows of cautery burns, using a bipolar cautery, are applied to the posterior wall of the incision in the scleral bed.

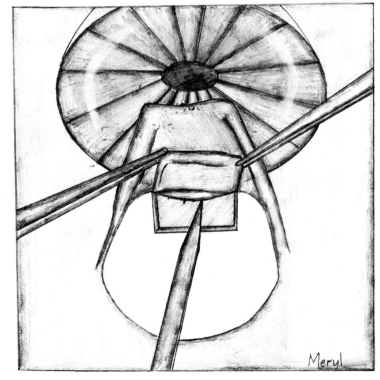

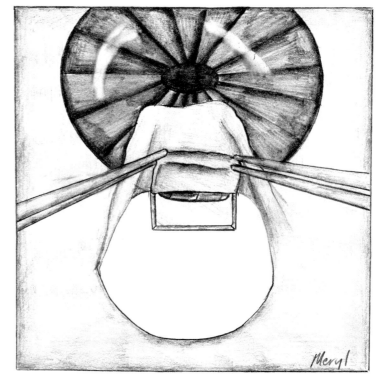

Figure 8.47. Subscleral Scheie (continued). The 4.5 mm long fistula is dissected into the anterior chamber. Iris prolapses into the incision.

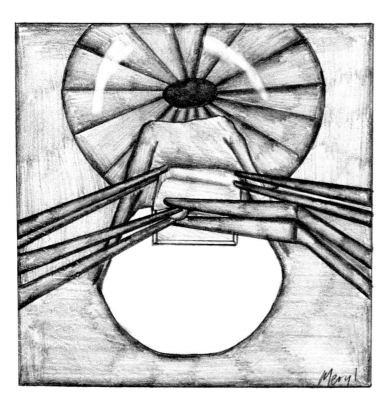

Figure 8.48. Subscleral Scheie (continued). A peripheral iridectomy is performed through the Scheie fistula.

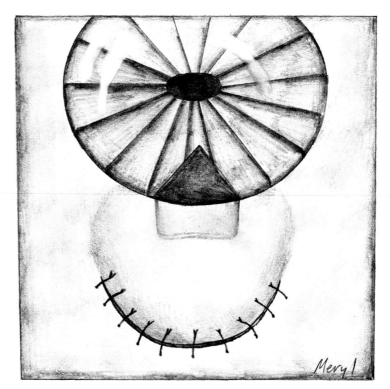

Figure 8.49. Subscleral Scheie (continued). The Tenon's capsule and conjunctival flap are separately sutured. The lamellar scleral flap is not sutured. Flow of aqueous through the fistula will push the lamellar scleral flap up against the conjunctiva.

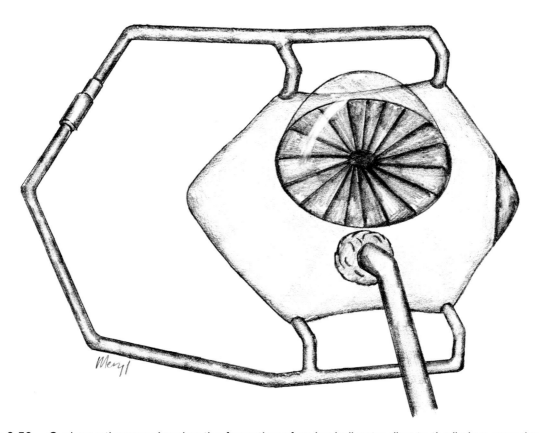

Figure 8.50. Cyclocryotherapy showing the formation of an ice ball extending to the limbus over the ciliary body.

CYCLOCRYOTHERAPY

The destruction of ciliary body tissue by using a freeze-thaw cycle can be effective in difficult cases on eyes that have a poor prognosis for other modes of surgery, e.g., refractory glaucoma in aphakic eyes or where repeated attempts to control intraocular pressure with other operations have failed. The effect, however, seems to be temporary, the drop in intraocular pressure persisting for 6 to 18 months. Care is needed to avoid excessive freezing, since destruction of too much ciliary body function can lead to phthisis. Conversely, insufficient freezing is ineffective. The main objection to the procedure is its unpredictability.

Technique

Usually local anesthesia is satisfactory. The operating microscope is not required for this procedure. A 3.0-mm retinal cryoprobe is used. This is applied over the ciliary body 3.5 mm from the limbus. It can be applied directly to sclera after raising a conjunctival flap but is more simply and as effectively done through conjunctiva and between the extraocular muscles, taking care not to injure an extraocular muscle. Two or three application sites are made in each quadrant of the globe.

Each application is a freeze-thaw cycle, freezing for 1 minute followed by thawing for 1 minute. The ice ball should just reach to the limbus without freezing the cornea (Fig. 8.50). This cycle may be repeated once or twice depending on whether two or three application sites are used and depending on the pressure-lowering effect required. When the intraocular pressure is high and the glaucoma has been refractory to treatment, a full hemisphere (two quadrants) can be treated at one sitting. It is better to undertreat at the first session and repeat the procedure in stages, rather than to risk overtreatment.

This operation is most useful as an adjunct procedure (1) after other operations, if the intraocular pressure is reduced but not adequately, e.g., intraocular pressure range 20 to 25 mm Hg; (2) as a final desperate measure when all other therapy for the glaucoma has failed, particularly in neovascular glaucoma and glaucoma in aphakic eyes.

Postoperative Treatment

Topical steroid drops are used until the postoperative uveitis is controlled.

Complications

See page 116.

Chapter 9

GLAUCOMA AND CATARACT

Senile cataract and primary open angle glaucoma or chronic angle closure glaucoma often coexist in the geriatric population and, with increasing longevity, are becoming more prevalent. The management of such cases has been controversial because medical or surgical therapy of one condition often affects the other (Maumenee and Wilkinson, 1970).

When cataract and glaucoma coexist but cataract extraction is not deemed necessary, the priority is to attempt medical control of the glaucoma without compromising vision. Medical therapy for glaucoma may include miotics, which may tend to reduce visual acuity regardless of pre-existing lens opacities and may cause an acceleration of cataract progression. Surgical therapy of glaucoma is also associated with increased lens opacification, especially if the surgery is complicated by hypotony or inadvertent lens trauma. Subsequent cataract extraction in an eye with glaucoma and a good functioning bleb results in loss of the bleb in 30 to 50% of eyes and inability to restore control of the glaucoma (Protonatarius et al., 1972; Rich, 1974; Wechsler and Robinson, 1980; Boyd, 1981). When the indications for cataract extraction are present but the glaucoma is controlled medically, the most common approach is to remove the cataract and continue medical management of the glaucoma. Intraocular pressure is more easily controlled in some eyes after lens extraction, but a significant number of these patients will require glaucoma surgery as early as 3 to 6 months after standard cataract extraction (Galin et al., 1961; Johnson, 1968; Bigger and Becker, 1971; Laatikainen, 1971; Linn, 1971; Randolph et al., 1971; Frankelson and Shaffer, 1974; Jerndal and Lundstrom, 1976). One is then faced with glaucoma surgery in an aphakic patient with a much poorer outlook (35 to 60%) for control of the intraocular pressure (Sugar, 1977; Luntz, 1979b). On the other hand, excellent results are reported with combined cataract extraction and trabeculectomy, where over 90% of eyes do well in terms of postoperative control of intraocular pressure with minimal risk of complications (Luntz and Berlin, 1980). These considerations favor some form of combined surgery when either the cataract or the glaucoma or both require surgery.

INDICATIONS FOR COMBINED SURGERY

The good results following combined surgery and the low risk of complications have led to a more aggressive use of this technique. The indications are:

1. Any eye with open angle glaucoma and cataract in which surgery is required for the cataract even if the glaucoma can be medically controlled with multiple medications. (If combined surgery is not done, many of these eyes will require glaucoma surgery at a later date. Glaucoma surgery in an aphakic eye has a poorer prognosis.)

2. An eye with uncontrolled open angle glaucoma requiring glaucoma surgery and with significant cataract with corrected vision of 20/40 or less (M. H. Luntz). A more conservative approach is favored by one of us (R. Harrison) when the visual acuity is better than 20/70 after pupil dilation.

Miotic therapy often reduces the potential vision when a cataract is present. A significant improvement in visual acuity is seen very often after simple trabeculectomy when the previously miotic pupil can be dilated even to a limited extent because the patient no longer requires miotics. On the other hand, there is some risk of progression of a cataract following any glaucoma operation. The status of the fellow eye must be considered. It is undesirable to produce unilateral aphakia by doing a combined operation when the fellow eye has adequate visual acuity and the patient is managing everyday tasks reasonably well. Improvement in extended wear soft contact lenses is making this problem less severe in some cases. When the fellow eye is already aphakic with a good visual result, it would be logical to be more radical in approach and carry out a combined cataract extraction with trabeculectomy and thus restore binocularity. This would also be applicable when the fellow eye has a cataract requiring extraction in the near future, with or without combined glaucoma drainage surgery.

COMBINED PROCEDURE FOR CATARACT-GLAUCOMA

Historically, cataract extraction has been combined with iridencleisis, trephination, sclerectomy, thermal sclerostomy and trabeculectomy (Wenaas and Stertzbach, 1955; Maumenee and Wilkinson, 1970; Laatikainen, 1971; Liaricos and Chilaris, 1973; Eustace and Harun, 1974; Frankelson and Shaffer, 1974; Francois, 1978; Johns and Layden, 1979). In these operations filtering procedures are combined with cataract extractions. All have the problem of attempting to produce satisfactory cataract wound closure and a filtering wound at the same time (Maumenee and Wilkinson, 1970; Frankelson and Shaffer, 1974; Francois, 1978; Johns and Layden, 1979). Cyclodialysis and trabeculotomy have also been combined with cataract extraction with varied success (Harrington, 1966; Galin et al., 1969; McPherson, 1976). Controversy regarding combined procedures arises in justifying a planned inadequate wound closure with the resultant possibility of postoperative complications related to shallow or flat anterior chamber.

Trabeculectomy is a safe and effective antiglaucoma operation (Cairns, 1968; Luntz, 1980) and is associated with fewer complications than the classical filtering procedures. When combined with cataract extraction, however, standard trabeculectomy, in which the lamellar scleral flap is left unsutured or loosely sutured, offers no advantage over other procedures regarding intraocular pressure control or complications stemming from inadequate closure of the wound (Liaricos and Chilaris, 1973; Eustace and Harun, 1974; Jerndal and Lundstrom, 1976; Witmer and Rohan, 1976; Johns and Layden, 1979). Suturing the scleral flap, however, will produce adequate wound closure and subsequently reduce these complications. Using this method, excellent control of glaucoma is obtained in approximately 90% of cases of trabeculectomy with cataract extraction. The results are far superior to trabeculectomy or any filtering operation in aphakic eyes. Trabeculotomy has its advocates, but our preference is trabeculectomy carried out with the standard limbal-based conjunctival flap (R. Harrison) or with a fornix-based conjunctival flap (M. H. Luntz). The trabeculectomy may also be

performed as an initial step followed by extraction through a corneal incision. Implantation of an intraocular lens can be done with combined glaucoma and cataract surgery but should be approached with caution since further glaucoma drainage surgery may be necessary in the future.

With appropriate indications, this modification of trabeculectomy combined with cataract extraction is the recommended therapy for concurrent senile cataract and primary open angle glaucoma or chronic angle closure glaucoma.

Preoperative Preparation

Preoperative treatment consists of lowering the intraocular pressure with intravenous mannitol (1.5 gm per kg of body weight). Topical hypotensive therapy should be withdrawn 24 hours before surgery because (1) pilocarpine will prevent adequate dilatation of the pupil for cataract extraction; (2) Timoptic and Diamox reduce aqueous formation and inhibit adequate bleb formation; and (3) adrenalin (epinephrine) derivatives may cause hypertension during the surgical procedure.

Topical steroids (prednisolone 1% q.i.d.) are introduced 1 day prior to surgery. Systemic indomethacin, 25 mg t.i.d. started 24 hours before surgery and continuing for 1 week after the surgery, may reduce postoperative inflammation and the incidence of cystoid macular edema. Postoperative treatment is similar to that of standard trabeculectomy.

Surgical Technique (Luntz and Berlin, 1980)

The operation is performed with the aid of an operating microscope under general anesthesia. The same magnifications are used for the difficult stages of the operation as in trabeculectomy.

CONJUNCTIVAL FLAP (5× to 7× MAGNIFICATION)

A fornix-based conjunctival flap is created extending 135 degrees at the superior limbus (14 mm). The conjunctiva is dissected posteriorly in the surgical plane between the conjunctiva/Tenon's capsule and the sclera (Fig. 9.1). Bleeding is controlled with cautery.

SCLERAL FLAP AND GROOVE FOR CATARACT INCISION (7× to 10× MAGNIFICATION)

In the center of the exposed sclera, a bipolar cautery is used to mark out a 3 mm × 3 mm trabeculectomy scleral flap hinged at the limbus. The radial lines of this flap are continued circumferentially at the limbus to create a 160 degree cataract incision just behind the "blue line" of the

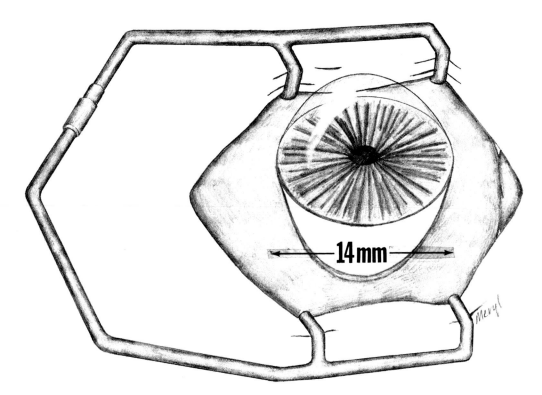

Figure 9.1. Cataract and trabeculectomy. A fornix-based conjunctival flap is created similar to the trabeculectomy flap, but extending 130 degrees (14 mm) at the superior limbus. The flap is dissected posteriorly in the surgical plane between Tenon's capsule and sclera.

surgical limbus, that is, in the scleral portion of the surgical limbus (Fig. 9.2).

Using either an oscillating knife, a diamond knife, a #75 Beaver knife or a disposable "superblade," a one-half thickness scleral groove is dissected along the cauterized line (Fig. 9.2). The cataract incision should be placed asymmetrically on each side of the trabeculectomy scleral flap by 10 degrees so that the longer incision is on the same side as the surgeon is "handed," thus facilitating lens delivery. The posterior incision of the 3 mm × 3 mm scleral flap is dissected to the level of the choroid, allowing an estimation of the thickness of the sclera (Fig. 9.3). The thickness chosen for the scleral flap depends on the pathology and the prognosis for surgery. Ideally, the flap should be one-third the scleral thickness, permitting adequate aqueous filtration and avoiding a very thin scleral flap which may become staphylomatous (Figs. 9.3 and 9.4). The scleral flap is dissected from the posterior incision at the desired thickness forward to just within the surgical limbus (Fig. 9.5)

TRABECULECTOMY (10× MAGNIFICATION)

Under the scleral flap, the salient external landmarks are easily discerned in the undissected scleral bed, as already described for trabeculectomy—

transparent deep corneal tissue, gray trabecular band, scleral spur and white, opaque sclera (Fig. 9.5).

A 2 × 2 mm square of cornea and trabecular zone is outlined deep to the scleral flap with its posterior border at the scleral spur (Fig. 9.5). The anterior border of the flap is incised to half the depth of the cornea followed by similar incisions at the sides (Fig. 9.6). With the internal flap outlined, the anterior chamber is entered at the anterior incision. Vannas scissors are carefully introduced and the anterior incision completed, without losing the anterior chamber (Fig. 9.7). The sides are incised to the scleral spur, and the internal corneo-trabecular block of tissue is removed by an incision just anterior to the scleral spur (Fig. 9.8). During this entire dissection the anterior chamber remains formed as the iris follows the scissors to block the opening (Fig. 9.9). Preplaced 10-0 nylon anchoring sutures at each corner of the lamellar scleral flap and posterior corners of the scleral dissection are inserted and moved out of the way (Fig. 9.10).

IRIDECTOMY (10× MAGNIFICATION)

A peripheral iridectomy, wider than the trabeculectomy, is made so that the marginal iris pillars cannot occlude the trabeculectomy opening

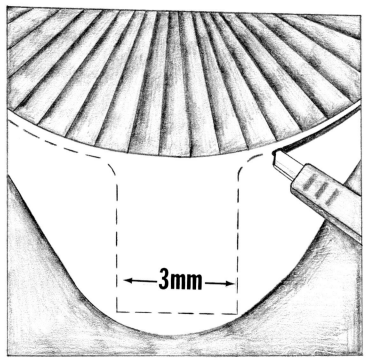

Figure 9.2. Cataract and trabeculectomy (continued). A 160 degree cataract incision, which includes a 3 mm × 3 mm scleral flap for the trabeculectomy dissection, is outlined by bipolar cautery. Dissection of the cataract-trabeculectomy incision is commenced with a diamond or a #74 Beaver blade knife at one end of the preplanned incision.

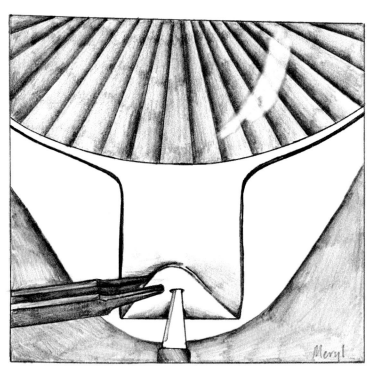

Figure 9.3. Cataract and trabeculectomy (continued). Dissection of the cataract-trabeculectomy flap is completed. The dissection extends to approximately half the scleral depth. The cataract incision can be placed asymmetrically by 10 degrees on each side of the trabeculectomy scleral flap with the longer incision on the same side as the surgeon is handed, facilitating lens delivery. Dissection of the trabeculectomy flap is commenced at one-third scleral thickness using a #74 Beaver blade.

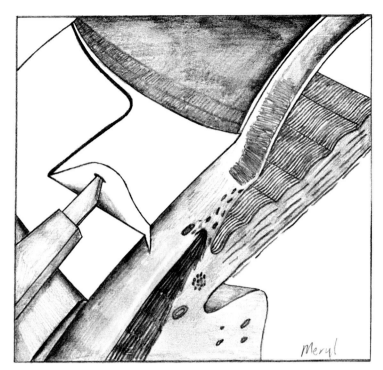

Figure 9.4. Cataract and trabeculectomy (continued). The cataract-trabeculectomy flap has been dissected, and the posterior incision is dissected down to the surface of the pars plana. The scleral thickness is estimated, and the dissection of the trabeculectomy flap is commenced in a surgical plane situated at one-third the thickness of the sclera so that the lamellar scleral flap is one-third the scleral thickness.

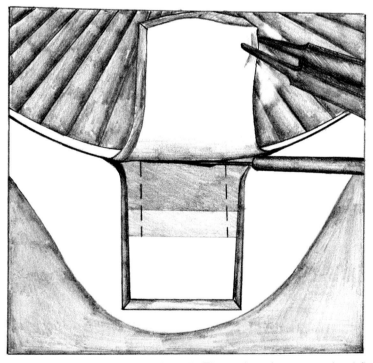

Figure 9.5. Cataract and trabeculectomy (continued). The trabeculectomy scleral flap is dissected to just within the surgical limbus. Under the scleral flap, the salient external landmarks are discerned in the undissected scleral bed with corneal tissue anteriorly, behind that a blue-gray band which is the external landmark for the trabecular meshwork, and the junction of the posterior limit of the trabecular zone with the sclera represents the external landmark for the scleral spur and the canal of Schlemm.

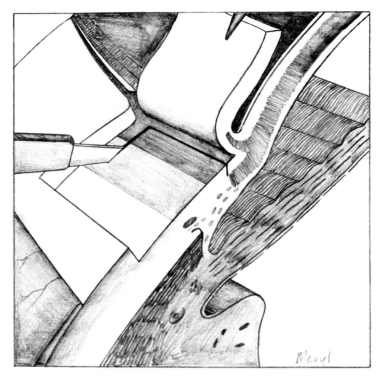

Figure 9.6. Cataract and trabeculectomy (continued). A 2 mm × 2 mm square of cornea and trabeculum is outlined in the deep scleral bed which represents the trabeculectomy opening. This is done exactly the same way as that described for trabeculectomy in Chapter 8.

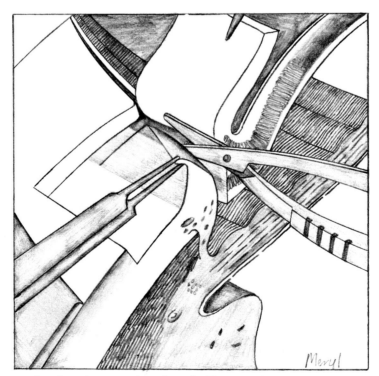

Figure 9.7. Cataract and trabeculectomy (continued). The anterior chamber is entered by dissecting an opening through the anterior incision of the trabeculectomy flap using a #74 Beaver blade. Vannas scissors are introduced, and the anterior incision is completed without losing the anterior chamber.

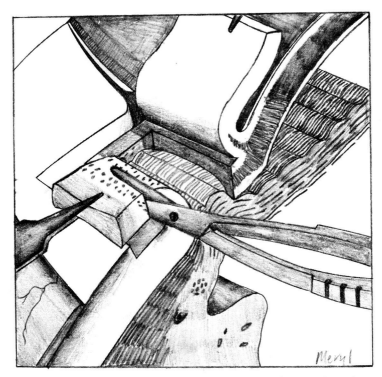

Figure 9.8. Cataract and trabeculectomy (continued). The sides of the trabeculectomy flap are cut to the scleral spur in the same way as described for trabeculectomy. The internal corneal-trabecular meshwork block of tissue so dissected is folded over and removed with an incision just anterior to the scleral spur.

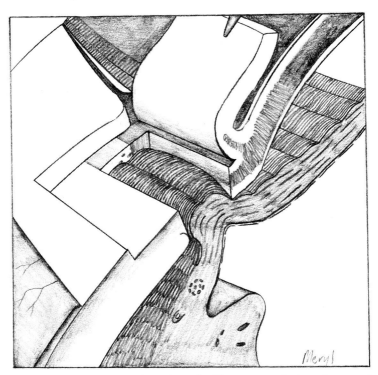

Figure 9.9. Cataract and trabeculectomy (continued). The cornea-trabecular meshwork block has been removed. Note how iris blocks the trabeculectomy opening so that the anterior chamber is maintained.

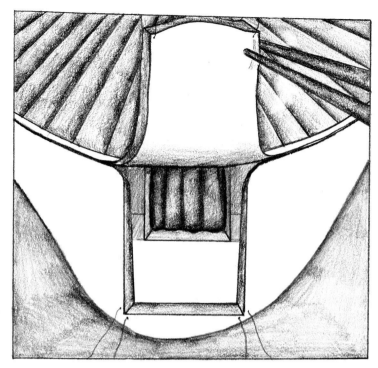

Figure 9.10. Cataract and trabeculectomy (continued). Diagram indicating surgeon's view of completed trabeculectomy. The lamellar scleral flap rotated forward onto the cornea is within the grooved incision made in preparation for the cataract incision. The trabeculectomy opening is shown within the lamellar scleral bed. Iris is visible plugging the trabeculectomy opening. The trabeculectomy opening extends back to the scleral spur; on each side is a narrow platform of deep corneal lamellae, and behind that is a trabecular band extending to the scleral spur. Behind the trabeculectomy opening and scleral spur are deep scleral lamellae. A 10-0 nylon suture is placed from each corner of the lamellar scleral flap to the posterior corners of the lamellar bed, and the sutures are moved out of the way.

postoperatively (Figs. 9.11 and 9.12). This iris is grasped with forceps, stretched to the right side and cut from the left (Fig. 9.11). The iridectomy is completed by cutting across the iris from the right side (Fig. 9.12).

CATARACT INCISION (10× MAGNIFICATION)

Corneal cataract scissors are introduced through the trabeculectomy opening (Fig. 9.13). With the deep blade in the anterior chamber, avoiding the iris, and the outer blade following the previously dissected limbal groove, the cataract incision is completed on each side of the trabeculectomy opening. Dissection of the cataract incision with knife and scissors as described will yield a smooth vertical cut with a bevel on the cornea facing the scleral side of the incision (Fig. 9.14).

PREPLACED SUTURES (10× MAGNIFICATION)

Two additional 10-0 nylon sutures are placed across the cataract incision precisely at the junction of the trabeculectomy flap at the limbus and the cataract incision. These sutures run obliquely at 45 degrees to the radial incisions of the scleral flap, are placed just anterior to Descemet's membrane on the corneal side and are full thickness in the sclera. They ensure correct apposition of the cataract incision after lens removal.

The sutures are looped away from the incision and the cornea lifted by grasping the trabeculectomy flap, opening the anterior chamber. Note that the base of the iridectomy is wider than the trabeculectomy (Fig. 9.14).

SEPARATION IRIS ADHESIONS (7× to 10× MAGNIFICATION)

The iris and pupil are inspected for posterior synechiae. If there are no synechiae or if there are only pigment adhesions to the lens capsule, the iris will move freely over the lens capsule. Absence of free movement of the iris indicates fibrous adhesions to the lens capsule, and mechanical separation is necessary. A round or flat iris spatula is introduced anterior to the iris surface and then under the iris through the pupil (Fig. 9.15), not through the iridectomy, sweeping from the pupil to the

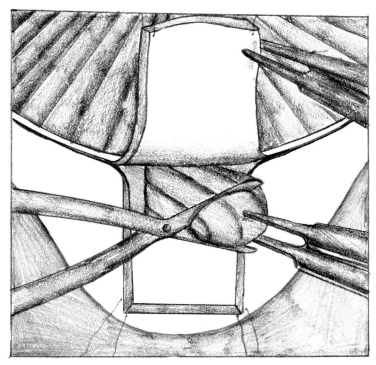

Figure 9.11. Cataract and trabeculectomy (continued). The iridectomy is made in the same way as that described for the trabeculectomy operation. The iris is grasped in the center of the trabeculectomy opening, pulled out of the trabeculectomy opening and moved first to the surgeon's right, putting the left pillar on stretch. Using an iridectomy scissor, the incision is half completed.

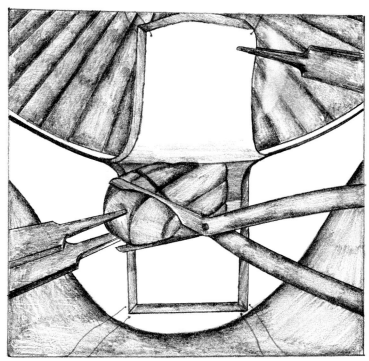

Figure 9.12. Cataract and trabeculectomy (continued). The iridectomy is completed by moving the iris across to the surgeon's left, putting the right pillar on stretch and completing the iridectomy. An alternative technique is described on page 68.

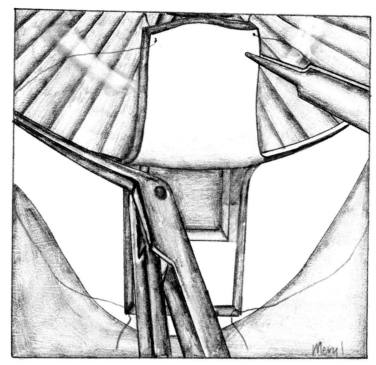

Figure 9.13. Cataract and trabeculectomy (continued). Standard microsurgical corneal cataract scissors are now introduced through the trabeculectomy opening, and, with the deep blade in the anterior chamber in front of the iris, the dissection of the cataract incision is completed on each side of the trabeculectomy opening.

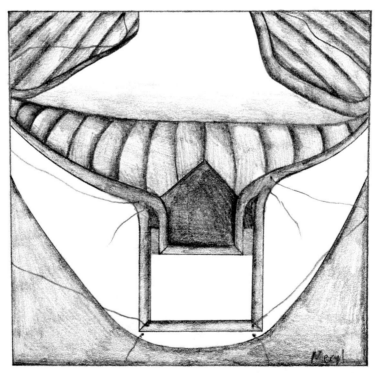

Figure 9.14. Cataract and trabeculectomy (continued). Dissecting the cataract incision in this way produces a smooth, vertical, 160 degree cataract incision with a deep bevel on the cornea facing the scleral side of the incision. Two additional 10-0 nylon sutures are placed across the cataract incision precisely at the junction of the trabeculectomy flap at the limbus and the cataract incision. These run obliquely at 45 degrees and are placed deeply in the incision. They are looped out of the way. Note that the iridectomy is larger than the trabeculectomy opening.

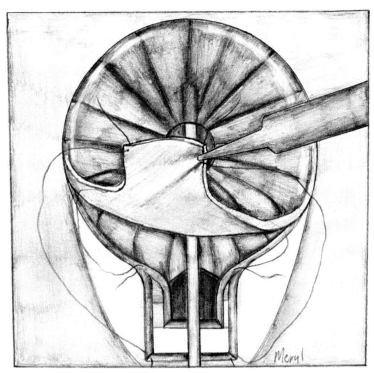

Figure 9.15. Cataract and trabeculectomy (continued). To correct posterior synechiae which are often present in these cases, an iris spatula coated with Healon is introduced in front of the iris as far as the pupil and then under the iris once it crosses the pupil.

periphery (Fig. 9.16). With this maneuver, synechiae are broken and pigment debris loosened by the spatula is swept under the iris and not into the pupil, thus maintaining a clear pupil. Note that the spatula does not enter through the iridectomy to reach the pupil. If this is done, debris and pigment are swept into the pupil.

An attempt is now made to open the pupil by placing a Weck sponge on the iris at the pupil margin and pulling toward the incision. If the pupil does not dilate because of fibrous tissue within the pupillary margin of the iris, one or more sphincterotomies are necessary. This is accomplished with Vannas scissors or Sutherland anterior segment scissors (Grieshaber), incising only half the width of the sphincter muscle (Fig. 9.17). The anterior surface of the scissors should be coated with Healon or the anterior chamber should be filled with Healon before introducing the scissors. Two inferior sphincterotomies are usually sufficient to allow extraction of the lens. An alternative approach is to make a radial incision from the tip of the peripheral iridectomy through the sphincter using Sutherland scissors, maintaining the anterior chamber with balanced salt solution. The lens is extracted through the sector iris opening so created. Following extraction of the lens, the radial iris incision is sutured with two interrupted sutures of 10-0 nylon

or 10-0 Prolene, one at the pupil margin and one placed at the opening of the peripheral iridectomy. Sphincterotomies give a better cosmetic result in the long run. The iris tends to atrophy where it is sutured, resulting in a pear-shaped pupil, whereas sphincterotomy retains a functional pupil.

CATARACT EXTRACTION (5× MAGNIFICATION)

Cryoprobe lens extraction is performed by the reverse tumbling technique (Fig. 9.18) followed by iris repositioning as required.

CLOSURE (10× MAGNIFICATION)

The two sutures at the posterior corners of the trabeculectomy flap are secured, followed by those at the limbus. Six additional interrupted 10-0 nylon sutures are placed to close the cataract incision. These sutures reach to Descemet's membrane on the corneal side of the incision and full depth in the sclera. They are secured only tightly enough to appose the wound edges. Too tight closure will induce postoperative astigmatism.

Closure of the trabeculectomy scleral flap is completed by two additional 10-0 nylon sutures on each side, halfway along the flap. A total of six interrupted sutures are used to close the trabeculectomy scleral flap, and six interrupted sutures are used to close the cataract incision (Fig. 9.19). The result is

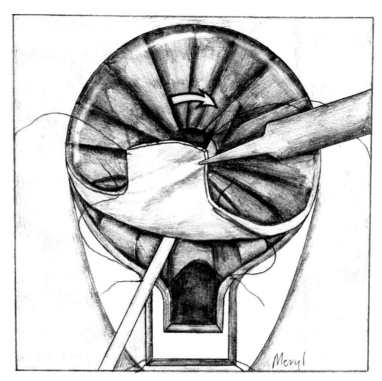

Figure 9.16. Cataract and trabeculectomy (continued). The spatula sweeps from the pupil to the periphery, thus breaking synechiae and moving any pigment debris under the iris rather than into the pupil.

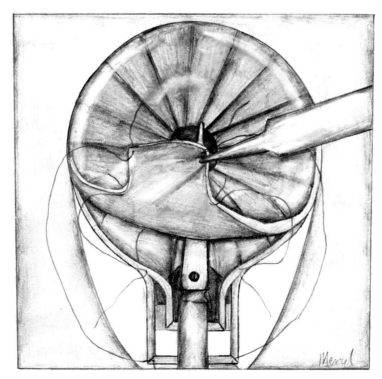

Figure 9.17. Cataract and trabeculectomy (continued). If there is fibrous tissue at the pupillary surface of the iris so that the pupil does not dilate, then one or more sphincterotomies should be performed. A Vannas scissors is introduced, performing one or more sphincterotomies in the lower portion of the pupil. Coating the anterior surface of the scissor with Healon will protect the corneal endothelium.

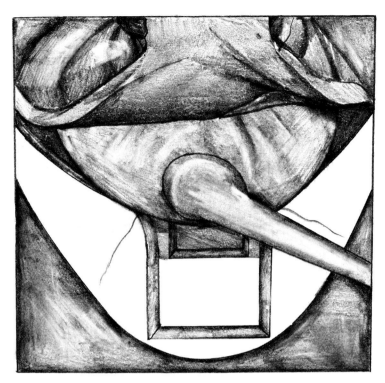

Figure 9.18. Cataract and trabeculectomy (continued). The lens is removed with a cryoprobe using a sliding or reverse tumbling technique.

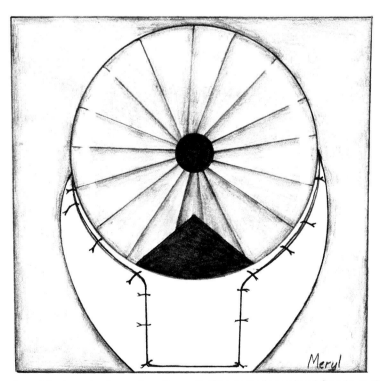

Figure 9.19. Cataract and trabeculectomy (continued). The lamellar scleral flap is replaced in position. The preplaced sutures have been tied, and the flap is closed with a total of six interrupted 10-0 nylon sutures. Good closure of the flap prevents postoperative shallow or flat anterior chambers. The cataract incision is closed with an additional three interrupted, deeply placed 10-0 nylon sutures at each side of the trabeculectomy, for a total of 14 sutures. Miochol has been used to constrict the pupil.

watertight wound closure, and a shallow or flat anterior chamber in the postoperative period is unlikely. The scleral flap adequately controls the flow of aqueous from the anterior chamber and prevents the formation of a staphyloma.

The conjunctiva is repositioned at the limbus and sutured with two interrupted 10-0 nylon sutures, securing the conjunctiva to the sclera at each end of the conjunctival flap and ensuring that the conjunctival edge lies snugly along the limbus (Fig. 9.20). Additional sutures may be placed from the conjunctival edge to limbal episcleral tissue at each side of the trabeculectomy scleral flap.

Balanced salt solution is injected under the conjunctival flap to separate it from the sclera, forming a bleb.

NeoDecadron drops are instilled before applying a patch and shield. The patient leaves the operating table with an intact anterior chamber and a bleb overlying the trabeculectomy. Routine cataract postoperative care follows.

Results

Postoperative control of intraocular pressure is achieved in over 90% of eyes (Luntz and Berlin, 1980). The average drop in intraocular pressure is 12.5 mm Hg. Results of the operation are summarized in Table 9.1. In this series, 32% of eyes required postoperative topical medication for adequate control of the intraocular pressure. Subconjunctival filtering blebs are not invariably present in successfully operated eyes.

Complications

There should be few complications and no serious postoperative problems. In 54 operated eyes (Luntz and Berlin, 1980) transient shallowing of the anterior chamber lasting less than 3 days was noted in two eyes (4%). A small postoperative hyphema (one-eighth anterior chamber) was noted in three eyes (5.5%), resolving spontaneously. In two eyes

Table 9.1 Combined Cataract/Trabeculectomy, 1967–1976

Forty-six eyes were followed for 2+ years—average 3.5 years.

No. Eyes	Average IOP[a] Preop on R$_x$	Average IOP Postop	Average Drop in IOP
8	18	13 (no med)	5
38	26	17 (13 meds.) (32%)	12.5

[a] IOP, intraocular pressure; MED, postoperative topical medications.

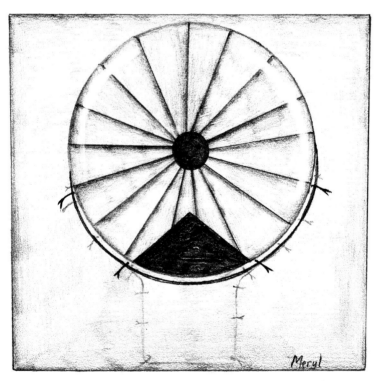

Figure 9.20. Cataract and trabeculectomy (continued). The conjunctival flap is rotated anteriorly to the limbus and sutured with two interrupted 10-0 nylon sutures at each end of the conjunctival flap so that it lies snugly along the limbus. Additional sutures may be placed from the conjunctival edge to the limbal episcleral tissue at each side of the trabeculectomy scleral flap.

(4%), intraocular pressure peaked above 21 mm Hg postoperatively with inadequate bleb formation. These patients did not sustain additional visual field loss in the follow-up period. These results indicate a very low risk of postoperative complications and excellent postoperative control of intraocular pressure when compared to other types of combined surgery reported in the literature.

Nevertheless, one author (R. Harrison) in 15 cataract extractions combined with a technique for trabeculectomy without multiple suturing of the scleral flap (see Chapter 8) encountered one eye which went into phthisis and one eye which had choroidal detachments due to massive hemorrhage within the suprachoroidal space. Vitreous may be pushed forward into the trabeculectomy opening, preventing drainage and resulting in a high intraocular pressure.

Reviewing the literature on postoperative complications in classifical filtering procedures (thermal sclerostomy, trephination, sclerectomy, iridencleisis) combined with cataract extraction reveals a higher incidence of postoperative complications than that observed with our technique. In the early series, steroids, trypsin, fine sutures and modern microsurgical techniques were, of course, not available (Birge, 1952; Wenaas and Stertzbach, 1955; Hughes, 1959; Hughes et al., 1963; Boberg-Ans, 1964; Harrington, 1966; Galin et al., 1969; Maumenee and Wilkinson, 1970; Liaricos and Chilaris, 1973; Eustace and Harun, 1974; Jerndal and Lundstrom, 1976; McPherson, 1976; Shields and Simmons, 1976; Witmer and Rohen, 1976; Johns and Layden, 1979).

Comparison of published reports of trabeculectomy using a loosely sutured or unsutured scleral flap combined with cataract extracton and of classical filtering procedures combined with cataract extraction reveals no significant statistical difference between the prevalence of postoperative complications, in particular the frequency of shallow or flat anterior chamber (Liaricos and Chilaris, 1973; Eustace and Harun, 1974; Jerndal and Lundstrom, 1976; Witmer and Rohen, 1976; Johns and Layden, 1979). The excellent postoperative results with respect to visual acuity improvement and intraocular pressure control in our cases and the low risk of postoperative complications compared to that observed in standard trabeculectomy and classical filtering procedures favor this technique. We emphasize, in particular, the importance of a tightly sutured scleral flap.

The high failure rate in cases treated with sequential rather than simultaneous surgery is also a strong argument for a combined procedure. This has motivated our less conservative approach to indications for surgery of either the cataract or the glaucoma.

Advantages of a Fornix-based Conjunctival Flap

There are a number of advantages to the use of a fornix-based conjunctival flap.

1. There is better exposure and visualization of the operative field. Dissection of the scleral flap into the cornea is facilitated. This ensures a trabeculectomy well anterior to the iris insertion and ciliary body and reduces the possibility of a hypertrophic ciliary body or iris adhesion obstructing the trabeculectomy opening.

2. The possibility of damaging the conjunctival flap during dissection, particularly "button-holing," is eliminated.

3. The procedure is technically easier than dissecting a limbus-based flap, especially when operating in an area of scarred conjunctiva from either previous trauma or surgery.

4. The well sutured scleral flap prevents excessive aqueous humor filtration and maintains the anterior chamber postoperatively. This explains the low incidence of postoperative shallow and flat anterior chambers when compared to classical filtering operations or trabeculectomy with loosely sutured (or presutured) scleral flap, combined with cataract surgery.

5. Suturing the scleral flap diminishes the risk of scleral staphyloma in cases of refractory glaucoma with high intraocular pressure (Spaeth and Rodriguez, 1977).

6. The fornix-based conjunctival flap adheres and scars to the limbus. As a result, the bleb forms posteriorly, producing a diffuse, well vascularized, thick-walled "low profile" bleb, well behind the limbus. There is less possibility of developing a thin, "high profile," avascular anterior bleb which overhangs the cornea, with the added risk of microscopic perforations of hypoxic conjunctiva and possible intraocular infection.

7. The posteriorly situated bleb allows safe early contact lens fitting, preferably with a soft extended wear lens. Our practice is to fit a Permalens as early as 2 weeks after the surgery.

INTRAOCULAR LENS IMPLANT

Glaucoma and cataract surgery simultaneously or separately performed may be combined with intraocular lens implantation if this is indicated. The indications for implanting an intraocular lens are the same in glaucoma patients as in nonglaucoma patients, although there are reservations which make this viewpoint controversial. Specific contraindications to implantation of an intraocular lens in a glaucoma patient are: (1) endothelial cell count less than 750 cells per mm^2, and (2) visual field within the 10 degree isopter over at least one quadrant with a large target.

A posterior chamber intraocular lens is preferable, and coating the lens with Healon before insertion into the anterior chamber is advantageous. The intraocular lens implant is inserted immediately after extracapsular removal of the cataract using the surgeon's standard technique for the extracapsular cataract extraction and implantation. The technique for doing an intraocular lens implantation is more difficult in glaucomatous eyes than in normal eyes due to prolonged miotic therapy causing small pupils which do not dilate well. When the pupil cannot be adequately dilated for extracapsular lens removal, multiple sphincterotomies are advantageous.

Chapter 10

MANAGEMENT OF SECONDARY GLAUCOMA

SURGICAL MANAGEMENT OF GLAUCOMA IN APHAKIC EYES

Glaucoma in the aphakic eye presents special problems in surgical management (Harrison R., in Sigelman and Jakobiec, 1984). Aphakic glaucoma is not a single nosological entity, for there are a wide variety of different mechanisms that cause glaucoma in the aphakic patient. It is more accurate to speak of glaucoma in the aphakic rather than aphakic glaucoma. The choice of treatment will, therefore, depend in part on the pathogenesis of the raised pressure. Not every eye with persistently raised intraocular pressure after cataract surgery needs to be treated. The decision to treat an eye either medically or surgically is based on the general indications for therapy:

1. Eyes with pathologic cupping of the disc and glaucomatous field loss.

2. Eyes with normal discs and visual fields with intraocular pressures persistently over 25 mm Hg in patients over 60 years of age. There is a high incidence of retinal vein occlusion in these eyes (David et al., 1977).

3. In eyes with normal discs and visual fields where surgical intervention is necessary for other reasons, e.g., vitreous strands adherent to the cataract section or corneo-vitreous touch with corneal endothelial decompensation.

To discuss adequately the surgical management of glaucoma in aphakia requires knowledge of the mechanisms which are causing the glaucoma. The mechanisms causing glaucoma in aphakic eyes have been comprehensively reviewed by Francois (1974). He quotes an incidence of between 1% and 7% following cataract operation, depending on the author. There is a higher incidence when chymotrypsin is used, which is similar to our experience. In most cases the glaucoma, unless present prior to cataract extraction, is the result of technical problems related to the cataract surgery and can often be prevented by detailed attention to the surgical technique at that time.

In a retrospective study of 1,014 eyes operated on for cataract (752 patients) and followed for a minimum of 12 months, 27 (2.6%) required treatment for raised intraocular pressure. Most of these eyes (81.5%) were successfully treated by medication alone and did not require surgery (Luntz, 1979b).

Types of Glaucoma in Aphakia

Glaucoma may predate the cataract extraction. Primary open angle glaucoma, angle closure glaucoma (whether an acute attack, repeated subacute attacks or chronic angle closure glaucoma with or without peripheral anterior synechiae) and secondary glaucomas may all produce post-cataract extraction glaucoma. Congenital, infantile and juvenile glaucomas in which the cataract may be an associated developmental anomaly or a complication of surgery for the glaucoma may also present high intraocular pressure following cataract extraction. Apart from certain specific circumstances, e.g., an intumescent cataract found with an acute angle closure glaucoma or the secondary glaucoma associated with a lens-induced uveitis, cataract extraction has an unpredictable effect on glaucoma. In open angle glaucoma sometimes the glaucoma is alleviated by the cataract extraction, but in many cases the glaucoma is not helped or may even become worse.

Prevention of Uncontrolled Glaucoma in Aphakia

Prevention of uncontrolled glaucoma in aphakia is better than attempting "cure." Unless the glaucoma is controlled with well tolerated and not excessive drug therapy prior to cataract extraction, appropriate therapeutic steps should be taken. In this respect, argon laser trabeculoplasty is promising to be a very valuable asset. Surgically, there are two options: (1) a combined trabeculectomy with cataract extraction; (2) a preliminary trabeculectomy followed by cataract extraction after an interval of about 2 months when postoperative inflammation has resolved. In this case, the extraction is best done through a corneal incision opposite the trabeculectomy site.

Mechanism of Glaucoma in Aphakia and Management

The mechanism of elevation of intraocular pressure in aphakia may be grouped into closed angle or open angle categories (see Table 10.1).

Glaucoma may present early in the first few days or some weeks or even months after cataract extraction.

SECONDARY ANGLE CLOSURE

Two main groups are recognized: (1) flat or shallow anterior chamber; (2) deep anterior chamber.

Angle Closure Glaucoma with a Flat or Shallow Anterior Chamber

A clinical presentation of a flat or shallow anterior chamber with a raised intraocular pressure falls within the definition of "malignant glaucoma," and

the mechanism may involve any one of the following:

Mechanisms

In the shallow anterior chamber group, the commonest cause of delayed reformation of the anterior chamber is pupil block. This may be associated with wound leakage and/or choroidal detachment and possibly ciliary body detachment. The intraocular pressure rises later and after the leak is sealed and peripheral anterior synechiae formation has occurred. More common predisposing factors for pupil block are inadequate or incomplete iridectomy, blood clot and/or vitreous block, intrapupillary pseudophakia, inflammatory reaction in which the iris and the vitreous face become adherent or membranous occlusion of the pupil. Posterior vitreous detachment also facilitates the forward movement of the intact anterior vitreous face to block the pupillary area. A third major cause of shallow anterior chamber is vitreous-ciliary block ("malignant glaucoma"). All these mechanisms can lead to the development of peripheral anterior synechiae. See Chapter 12, pages 127–131.

Treatment

Pupillary Block

Mydriatic therapy is carried out initially, using scopolamine 0.25% and phenylephrine 2.5%. This may abolish the pupillary block, and the anterior

Table 10.1 Permanent Glaucoma Mechanisms
Permanent glaucoma mechanisms after cataract extraction may be differentiated by gonioscopy. Common transient early glaucoma causes include tight wound closure, inflammatory reaction, alpha-chymotrypsin, and hyphema. Rare late causes are epithelial and fibrous ingrowth.

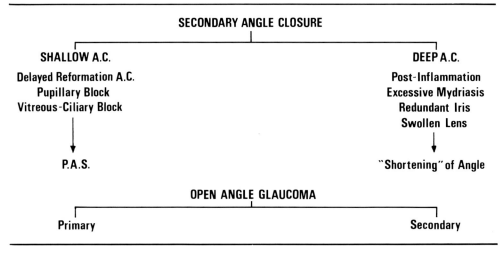

chamber promptly deepens. When mydriatics fail, a cure is usually achieved by an adequate peripheral iridectomy performed through the cornea superiorly or at the 6 o'clock position. Laser iridectomy may be attempted if the cornea is clear and the anterior chamber not too shallow, but if relief is not obtained early enough (within 48 to 72 hours if the anterior chamber is flat) extensive peripheral anterior synechiae formation will ensue.

A large air bubble can cause pupillary block within a day or two, especially when the iridectomy has been incomplete or is too small. The air may be confined to the anterior chamber, may partially pass into the posterior chamber in "collar stud" fashion or may be trapped entirely behind the iris. Angle closure is likely to ensue. This complication is rarely seen with a sector iridectomy or with multiple iridectomies. To abolish the block, the initial treatment is medical with mydriatics and hypotensive agents. The air bubble tends to absorb rapidly in a few days, and surgical removal of the air by paracentesis is not usually necessary.

Vitreous-Ciliary Block

Vitreous-ciliary block in aphakia does not respond to cycloplegic-mydriatic treatment as in the phakic eye. It rarely arises de novo after cataract extraction. Lens extraction alone does not cure a pre-existing malignant glaucoma. It is best treated by aspiration of posterior vitreous (see Chapter 12, pp. 132–138).

Angle Closure Glaucoma with a Formed Anterior Chamber—Mechanisms

Here the etiologic factors are excessive postoperative inflammatory reaction due to inadequate postoperative steroids, prolonged mydriasis usually due to excessive use of atropine over many weeks and a redundant iris, as seen commonly after an intumescent cataract has been present. Treatment with phospholine iodide is often successful. Timolol may be of supplementary value. Surgery is necessary if medical treatment fails (see below, "Selection of Surgical Procedure").

OPEN ANGLE GLAUCOMA IN APHAKIA

The second major category of postoperative glaucoma in aphakia is characterized by an open angle. The most frequent etiology is primary open angle glaucoma present before the cataract extraction. There may be preoperative confirmatory data of open angle glaucoma, and the fellow eye may have evidence of primary open angle glaucoma. In the absence of such confirmatory data, it is possible that primary open angle glaucoma may arise de novo in aphakia. This would be suspected if the fellow, phakic eye develops primary open angle glaucoma.

Secondary open angle glaucoma is due to chymotrypsin, steroids or particulate matter blocking the trabecular meshwork, e.g., vitreous, blood or blood products, ghost cells (ghost cell glaucoma), lens material (phakolytic glaucoma). Inflammatory reaction is an aggravating factor. In practice, it may be difficult to differentiate these various mechanisms, and the glaucoma may have multiple causative factors. Medical treatment is generally effective. The aphakic eye is more responsive to phospholine iodide than the phakic eye. Epinephrine agents are proven to cause maculopathy in 30% of eyes treated and must be used with caution in minimal dosage. Timolol and carbonic anhydrase inhibitors may be necessary. Surgical intervention is sometimes necessary, but the results of glaucoma surgery in aphakia are not as successful as in phakic eyes.

Alpha-Chymotrypsin

A transitory rise of intraocular pressure in seen in eyes following cataract surgery in which chymotrypsin is not used (at least 8% of eyes operated) with no definable cause and considerably higher in eyes in which chymotrypsin is used. The pressure rise from chymotrypsin is transitory, seen from the second or third day to the fifth day, and resolves spontaneously. Occasionally, the pressure elevation lasts 1 to 2 weeks. When the intraocular pressure is high enough to demand treatment, control is usually obtained with Timoptic, miotics and/or acetazolamide. Timoptic can be used prophylactically before and after the surgical procedure, particularly in patients with advanced visual field loss.

Transient Normal Postoperative Pressure Rise

In the first 24 hours after uncomplicated surgery without the use of trypsin, the high intraocular pressure is almost certainly related to accurate, watertight suturing of the corneo-scleral incision. Probably plasmoid aqueous plays a contributory part. It is also possible that deformation of the corneo-scleral area by the sutures may reduce outflow. This common pressure deviation accounts for the postoperative pain and requires treatment only with analgesics.

Vitreous

The presence of free vitreous in the anterior chamber is usually innocuous, especially when due to spontaneous breach of the anterior hyaloid after completion of uneventful cataract extraction. It may, however, cause elevated intraocular pressure. This is much more likely to occur when there has been intraoperative vitreous loss and inadequate vitrectomy. Residual lens cortex material is another cause of early glaucoma, especially when a large amount is present. Multiple causative factors may combine. Vitreous may be mixed with the lens cortical material, thus intensifying the problem. Hyphema and inflammatory reaction further exacerbate the glaucomatogenic conditions. Aspiration of the lens material and/or vitreous is best accomplished by a closed irrigation-aspiration-cutting system.

Hyphema

Hyphema usually originates from the iridectomy site and sometimes from the cataract incision. Small hyphemas are benign and absorb quickly. A large hyphema may be accompanied by a rise of intraocular pressure if enough of the angle is blocked and the remaining angle superiorly is functionally incompetent due to blockage of the trabecular meshwork by cellular material and debris after the lens extraction. Medical treatment, including hyperosmotic agents, usually suffices. Unrelieved glaucoma can cause blood staining of the cornea, rupture of the hyphema into vitreous, leading to ghost cell glaucoma later, and the development of peripheral anterior synechiae. These complications can be prevented by timely evacuation of the hyphema.

Evacuation of the Hyphema

Two paracentesis incisions are made at the posterior limbus, each under a small conjunctival flap, 180 degrees apart, generally at the 3 o'clock and 9 o'clock meridian. A 22-gauge needle attached to a pediatric intravenous set is inserted into the anterior chamber through the nasal parencentesis opening, and this is connected to a bottle of normal saline or Ringer's solution. The height of the bottle can be adjusted as it is suspended from a stand. The anterior chamber is constantly infused by gravity, and at the same time the inferior lip of the temporal paracentesis incision is depressed with a flat spatula, allowing blood to be washed out of the anterior chamber. If the blood does not flow out freely, an Ocutome can be introduced and the blood

carefully aspirated. This is particularly useful when the blood is mixed with lens material from a damaged lens and/or vitreous.

The blood may have clotted, making evacuation difficult or impossible. In these cases a few minims of urokinase are injected into the anterior chamber. After a few minutes the clot will lyse and can be aspirated out of the chamber.

When most of the blood is removed, any residual clots attached to the iris should not be disturbed. At this point, a careful inspection is made for any bleeding points on the iris or ciliary body; if found, they are cauterized using bipolar cautery. Air is left in the anterior chamber at the end of the procedure.

Steroid-induced Glaucoma

The use of topical steroids in the postoperative treatment will cause a steroid-induced glaucoma in susceptible individuals.

Characteristically, raised intraocular pressure occurs from the tenth to the fourteenth day after commencing topical steroids and rapidly reverts to normal if the steroids are withdrawn. This condition is often misdiagnosed and perpetuated by not curtailing the steroid treatment.

SELECTION OF SURGICAL PROCEDURE

Surgery is indicated if medical treatment fails to control the glaucoma or for other reasons, e.g., reconstruction of the anterior chamber after trauma. An impressive variety of operations have been described, mainly with disappointing or conflicting results. Cyclodialysis, once a popular operation for aphakic glaucoma, or cyclodialysis with angiodiathermy rarely gives a good long term result; only one-third or fewer of the operated eyes remain under control (Paufique and Sourdille, 1969; Sugar, 1977). D'Ermo (1975) claims good results with the irido-cycloretraction operation (see below), but Chavand et al. (1976) and Sugar (1977) using the same operation report very poor results. One of us (R. Harrison) has had some success with a modified form of this operation. Villon (1976) suggests cyclocryotherapy (see Chapter 8) in aphakic glaucoma but does not give detailed supportive results.

Technique of Cyclodialysis (5× to 7× Magnification)

The aim of cyclodialysis is to obtain a communication between the anterior chamber and the suprachoroidal space by separation of the ciliary body from its attachment to the scleral spur. In successful cases, gonioscopy shows a cleft in the angle at the site of the cyclodialysis. The success rate is no better than 25 to 40% including medical therapy. The chief indication is chronic open angle glaucoma in aphakia. Areas of angle vascularization should be avoided if possible. A superior quadrant is preferable to avoid a blood clot blocking the cyclodialysis cleft. The procedure is less effective if a vitreous mushroom occupies a major part of the anterior chamber.

Our technique is to perform a sclerotomy under a small limbus-based conjunctival flap down to the uveal tissue 5 mm posterior and parallel to the limbus for 3 mm in extent. A narrow cyclodialysis spatula is inserted radially until the tip is seen entering the anterior chamber. It is important to avoid perforating the ciliary body and causing hemorrhage in the vitreous as well as hyphema. The tip of the spatula is prevented from entering the posterior chamber by pressing it against the sclera in its passage forward and by keeping the heel of the instrument back against the sclera externally. Upon entering the anterior chamber, the tip is depressed slightly to avoid stripping Descemet's membrane. Two similar parallel insertions are made, and the narrow clefts are joined by lateral sweeping movements. A small hyphema is common. This procedure causes less bleeding than the classical Heine cyclodialysis in which a quadrant of ciliary body separation is obtained from one point of entry by making a fan-shaped sweep. Air injection into the anterior chamber along the cyclodialysis cleft is done only if bleeding is considerable. The air bubble may block further entry of blood into the anterior chamber. A period of low intraocular pressure for several days may suddenly lead to a steep elevation of pressure due to blockage of the cleft by a blood clot. Intravenous mannitol often relieves this blockage, and the pressure control is maintained. When osmotherapy fails, paracentesis of the anterior chamber may be curative. Postoperative treatment consists of steroid drops and a long acting miotic (Phospholine iodide).

Cyclodialysis is an obsolescent procedure because of its high failure rate, although it has the virtues of simplicity and lack of serious complications. Irido-cycloretraction offers a somewhat higher success rate, although it is far from satisfactory.

Technique of Cycloretraction (Modified from Krasnov; also Termed Irido-Cycloretraction) (5× to 7× Magnification)

The procedure is essentially a cyclodialysis with insertion of two scleral strips along the cyclodialysis cleft into the angle of the anterior chamber. The scleral strips act as mechanical obstacles to prevent closure of the cleft. The original operation as described by Krasnov consisted of forming two parallel scleral strips 5 mm long and 2 mm wide, cut at half the scleral thickness and hinged at 5 mm from the limbus. We have found the procedure best modified by (1) making the strips 6 mm in length to allow for shrinkage; (2) making the strips somewhat radial rather than parallel (Figs. 10.1 to 10.3). The cyclodialysis tracks are made from the sclerotomy at the hinges of the strips (Fig. 10.4), which are then inserted and thrust into the anterior chamber (Fig. 10.5). When visible in the anterior chamber, the inserted strips are impaled through the cornea with a micro needle to hold them in situ while withdrawing the forceps used for their introduction. Otherwise, the scleral strips tend to be withdrawn inadvertently. Air is not introduced into the anterior chamber. The conjunctival flap is sutured back with a continuous 8-0 Vicryl suture (Fig. 10.6). Cycloretraction is not advised when the vitreous face bulges into the anterior chamber since vitreous will block the cleft.

The only common complication is hyphema, which always absorbs in a few days. (We have encountered one case of malignant glaucoma which was cured by trabeculectomy with vitrectomy.) The results are about 60% successful, but supplementary medical therapy is usually necessary to obtain successful control. As with cyclodialysis, success is not always permanent.

Cyclocryotherapy (See Chapter 8)

When carefully performed to avoid the danger of phthisis from overdosage, cyclocryotherapy is useful as an adjunct procedure to reduce the preoperative pressure in the aphakic eye if it is very high (over 45 mm Hg) and present a less congested eye with less tendency for serious bleeding at the time of intraocular surgery. Cyclocryotherapy is more commonly carried out after the glaucoma surgery if the pressure has not fallen to an acceptable level. After cyclocryotherapy, permanent peripheral corneal edema has been noted. A permanent 3+ flare without cells is not uncommon. Choroidal and retinal exudative detachments have been encountered. Macular edema is well recognized. Hyphema is common, especially with neovascularization. Phthisis bulbi especially after repeated cyclocryotherapy has been described.

Our experience on the whole confirms the unsatisfactory results with these operations in aphakic

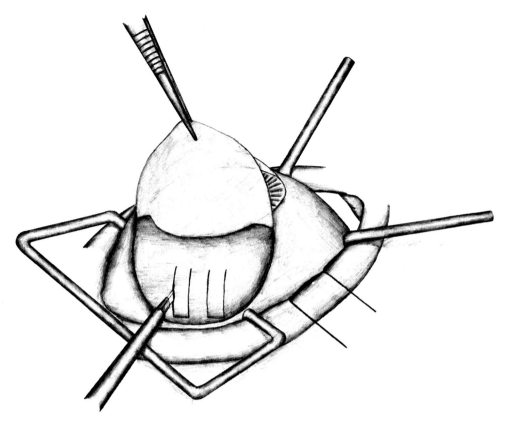

Figure 10.1. Cycloretraction. A limbus-based conjunctival-Tenon's flap is raised over the upper half of the eye (see discussion of trabeculectomy with limbus-based flap, Chapter 8, p. 72). Two radially placed scleral strips hinged at 5 mm from the limbus, 6 mm long and 2 mm wide, are cut at half the scleral thickness.

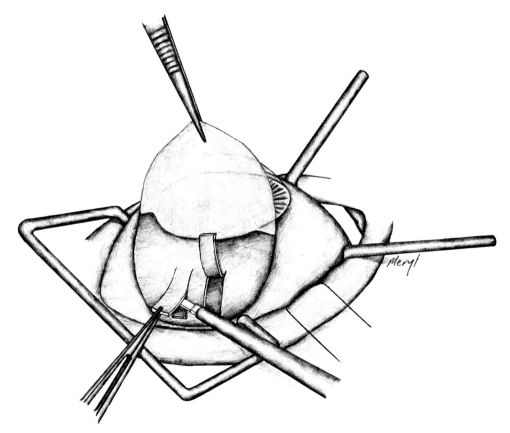

Figure 10.2. Cycloretraction (continued). The two scleral strips are dissected out at half the scleral thickness, hinging the strips 5 mm from the limbus.

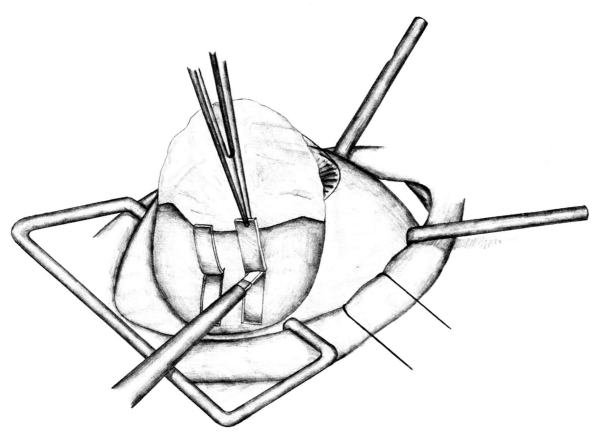

Figure 10.3. Cycloretraction (continued). Completion of the dissection of the two scleral strips. The sclera is dissected to the surface of the pars plana at the base of each strip.

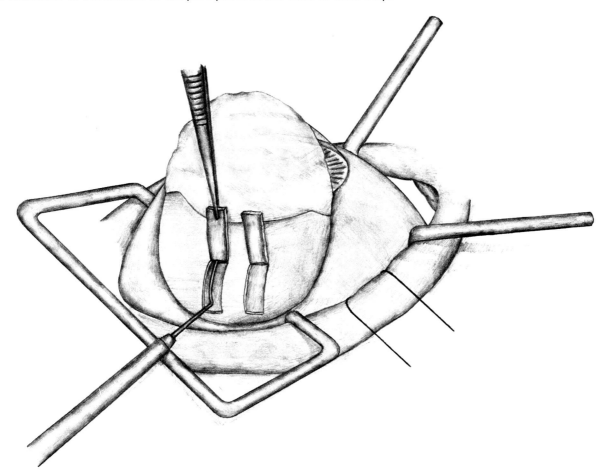

Figure 10.4. Cycloretraction (continued). A cyclodialysis spatula is introduced at the base of each strip, and a cyclodialysis tract is made from each strip by thrusting the spatula into the anterior chamber.

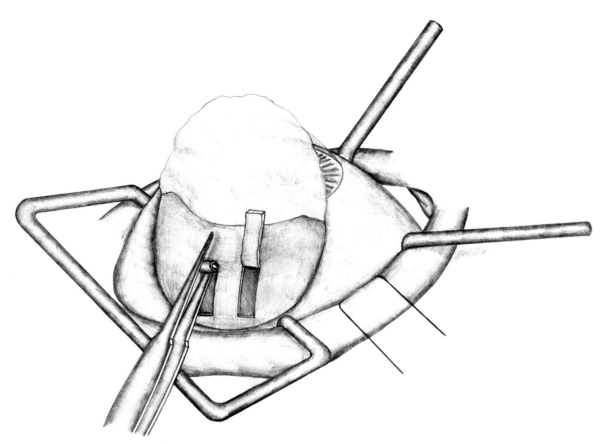

Figure 10.5. Cycloretraction (continued). Using a fine forceps, each strip is bent on itself and the free edge of the strip is introduced into the cyclodialysis track. The entire length of the strip is then fed into the cyclodialysis track and into the anterior chamber.

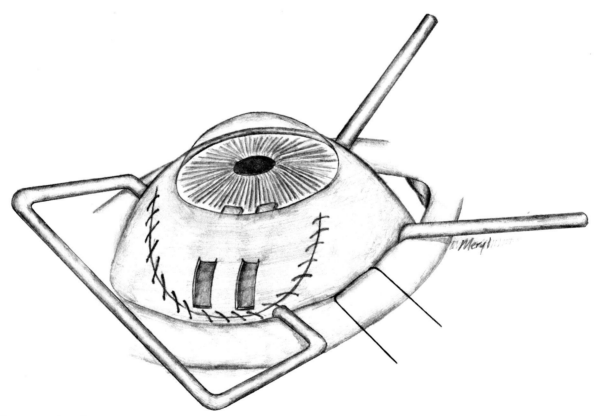

Figure 10.6. Cycloretraction (continued). The conjunctival flap is sutured back with a continuous 8-0 virgin silk suture. The free ends of the two strips are visible in the anterior chamber.

glaucomas. It has been difficult to obtain long term control of intraocular pressure with any of these procedures.

Subscleral Scheie with Anterior Vitrectomy

Our poor results with the previous procedures have led us to use subscleral Scheie combined with partial anterior vitrectomy as the primary operation in aphakic eyes with glaucoma, except those due to pupil block. The vitrectomy is mandatory. The operation has few complications. A standard subscleral Scheie technique is used (see Chapter 8). The vitrectomy is performed with a suction, cutting and infusion instrument system. This is done through a separate limbal incision after closing the conjunctival flap upon completion of the Scheie operation.

SECONDARY GLAUCOMA DUE TO UVEITIS

Uveitis can lead to secondary glaucoma due to inflammatory reaction blocking the trabecular meshwork, peripheral anterior synechiae formation and pupillary block. Judicious use of steroids postoperatively usually prevents uveitic glaucoma unless aggravating factors are also present.

Treatment

Treatment is medical in the first instance and emphasizes control of the uveitis. When and if the uveitis has resolved, the glaucoma will become controlled unless there is widespread trabecular fibrosis or chronic angle closure. Medical treatment follows a standard pattern:

1. Mydriatics, if there is an active uveitis. Phenylephrine (Neo-Synephrine) and Mydriacil are preferable to the use of Cyclogyl (cyclopentolate hydrochloride) or atropine derivatives because the former have less pharmacologic pressure-elevating effect.

2. Topical corticosteroids. Prednisolone, dexamethasone or betamethasone are preferred to fluoromethylone because the latter is a weak anti-inflammatory agent.

3. Systemic corticosteroids, if the uveitis is unusually severe. Prednisolone in doses of up to 120 mg daily or equivalent, monitored by the anterior chamber reaction.

4. In refractory cases, not responding to systemic and topical steroids, the use of systemic cytotoxic agents must be seriously considered, e.g., azathioprine, cyclophosphamide (Friedman et al., 1982). These have been used to gain control of the uveitis or to permit reduction of the dose of systemic steroids if very high doses have become necessary. Cytotoxic and immunosuppressive drugs, however, present dangerous side effects, including bone marrow depression, and must be used with great care.

Surgical Treatment of Secondary Open Angle Glaucoma from Uveitis

Surgery is indicated if an appropriate intraocular pressure is not achieved with medication, if there is noticeable enlargement of the cup to disc ratio or increasing visual field loss. Patients over 65 years of age with intraocular pressure over 26 mm Hg run a higher than usual risk of central or branch vein occlusion, and these patients should be operated on sooner. Careful consideration must be given to choosing the most appropriate surgical procedure, every effort having been made to achieve control of the uveitis before surgery is performed. In chronic uveitis a reaction of 1+ cells and flare is compatible with control of the disease.

Argon laser trabecular surgery should be the first choice if the uveitis is controlled and the eye is quiet. An average reduction of 10 mm Hg results in 70% of eyes operated on. The pressure-lowering effect of laser trabeculoplasty appears to correlate with the height of the initial intraocular pressure (see "Techniques of Laser Trabeculoplasty," Chapter 8).

Trabeculectomy in general will reduce intraocular pressure an average of 16 to 17 mm Hg, but the results in secondary glaucoma are slightly less successful when a reduction of 20 mm Hg is required. For example, when the pressure is over 40 mm Hg on full medication, then trabeculectomy is not likely to reduce the pressure to acceptable levels. In these cases, a subscleral Scheie operation is more efficacious.

The Subscleral Scheie operation is remarkably effective in secondary glaucomas and if properly performed has few complications, although the risk of complications is higher than with trabeculectomy (see Chapter 8). It is the operation of choice in eyes in which the uveitis is still active, or if the intraocular pressure needs to be lowered by more than 20 mm Hg or in cases where trabeculectomy has failed. In the event these operations fail repeatedly, cyclocryotherapy may be done as a last measure or a seton may be resorted to (see Chapter 11). Pigmentary glaucoma and pigment dispersion syndrome can be regarded as secondary glaucomas but are dealt with as primary glaucomas.

GLAUCOMA SURGERY FOLLOWING PENETRATING KERATOPLASTY

Pupil Block

In all cases of glaucoma following keratoplasty, the pupil should be dilated for the first week to exclude a pupil block mechanism. This can arise from excessive filtering through the transplant incision and crowding in the anterior chamber angle. When a mydriatic controls the intraocular pressure, no further treatment is required. The incidence of postoperative glaucoma is lower if the donor button is larger than the recipient opening. This is possibly the result of a deeper anterior chamber and easier access of aqueous to the normal outflow system.

Surgical Treatment

Only if medical treatment fails after 6 to 8 weeks to reduce intraocular pressure to less than 25 mm Hg and particularly if the cornea becomes decompensated, surgical treatment is indicated. The surgical treatment for this type of secondary glaucoma is difficult, especially when the peripheral iris and host cornea become fused after prolonged contact, thus obliterating the angle.

TRABECULECTOMY

A trabeculectomy is the operation of choice and in many cases will cure the condition. The success rate for control of intraocular pressure is in the region of 65 to 75%—not as high as in primary open angle glaucoma. If the eye is aphakic, a trabeculectomy or subscleral Scheie with anterior vitrectomy should be performed (see Chapter 8). Trabeculectomy can be repeated in another quadrant if unsuccessful, or, preferably, a subscleral Scheie should be performed.

When two such attempts at filtration have failed, it is unlikely that a third will be successful. Cyclocryotherapy should then be done. Cyclocryotherapy, even as an initial procedure, is valuable in eyes in which extensive formation of anterior synechiae to the donor and host cornea has obliterated the anterior chamber. This procedure generally controls intraocular pressure although often for only a limited period of time.

Surgery for secondary glaucoma following penetrating keratoplasty should be postponed as long as possible because approximately 30% of clear grafts become opaque as a result of glaucoma surgery.

Chapter 11

ALLOPLASTIC DEVICES IN GLAUCOMA SURGERY: SETONS

Many foreign materials designed to aid drainage in glaucoma surgery have been implanted for the past 75 or so years in both human and animal eyes. The first setons were made of horse hair. Silk thread, nylon, gelatin film, silicone, tubes made from plastic, metallic insertions of gold, platinum, tantalum, gold-molybdenum alloy and bundles of stainless steel wires have all been implanted (Krejci et al., 1970). On the whole, these alloplastic devices have not withstood the test of time and have disappeared from use and from current literature because of a high incidence of complications and failure. They have predominantly been replaced by translimbal tubes extending from the anterior chamber to the subconjunctival space. In many instances they have maintained the scleral opening and acted as a "wick" to promote flow of aqueous through the fistula. In spite of good drainage and the formation of a large bleb in the early postoperative period, later foreign body reaction leads to bleb shrinkage and drainage virtually ceases after 4 to 6 weeks in spite of an often patent fistula. This end result is consistent with the experience of most glaucoma surgeons that exploration of a failed filtering site generally reveals a patent scleral fistula but a fibrosed bleb. Thus, successful filtration surgery depends more on maintaining a functional bleb than on maintaining a functioning fistula. As most setons have been devices to maintain a functioning fistula, these have often failed for the same reason that glaucoma filtering surgery fails. Some seton procedures have failed because of extrusion and some because of prolonged hypotony.

Three different plastic implants have, however, given encouraging results and are still being used in patients with failed glaucoma surgery and by some surgeons as an initial procedure in patients with neovascular glaucoma. In our view, these al-loplastic devices should not be used in any patient, including those with neovascular glaucoma, until one or more standard filtration procedures have failed. There is no sound evidence that these devices give better results as the initial procedure in any form of glaucoma, including neovascular glaucoma. We have already described a method for modified trabeculectomy in cases of neovascular glaucoma, and this should be tried as the initial procedure for that condition.

It is our practice to attempt at least two, rarely three, filtering procedures; if these measures fail, we then proceed to the use of an alloplastic device. In neovascular glaucoma, however, it is acceptable to proceed to a seton device as the second procedure.

The three techniques that are still used are based on those described by Molteno et al. (1979), that described by Krejci et al. (1970) in animals and subsequently in humans (Krejci, 1980) and more recently the technique described by Krupin et al. (1980).

TECHNIQUE FOR SETON INPLANTATION

This method, described in 1969 (Molteno and Luntz), utilizes a prosthesis made from methylmethacrylate and designed in two parts. A flat plate was fashioned to conform to the sclera, approximately circular in shape and 8.5 mm in diameter. The radius of curvature of the undersurface was approximately 11.5 mm. The anterior two-thirds of the plate was faceted on its upper surface so that the thickness of the plate varied from 0.15 mm anteriorly to 1.0 mm at its posterior edge. This design was intended to prevent Tenon's capsule and conjunctiva from shrinking onto the scleral surface and obliterating the bleb. A gutter was incorporated at the junction with the translimbal tube to assure an even spread of aqueous drainage into the bleb. A translimbal tube 1.0 mm in length with an external diameter of 1.5 mm and an internal diameter of 0.75 mm was fixed to the anterior part of the plate and inserted into the scleral fistula. The plate was sutured to the sclera.

Our initial study reported results of the operation in 31 eyes with advanced glaucoma in which two or three standard glaucoma operations had failed. We were able to control the pressure in 26 eyes (87%) with few complications.

These encouraging results led to further improvements in the design of the prosthesis and the surgical technique (Molteno et al., 1979). The present prosthesis is designed with a biconcave base plate (silicone) which rests on the sclera and a long silicone tube (Figs. 11.1 and 11.2). A major change in design involves the tube, which has been lengthened considerably (Fig. 11.1). Recently, there has been increasing interest in alloplastic devices for glaucoma surgery, particularly for neovascular glaucoma, which has led to a resurgence in the use of this procedure.

Technique

PREPARATION

The patient is prepared and draped in the standard sterile manner. Akinesia and anesthesia are obtained with a local injection of Xylocaine 1.5% with epinephrine 1:200,000 in a Van Lint fashion and a retrobulbar injection of Xylocaine 1.5% with Wydase.

With the microscope in position, a lid speculum is inserted and the eye is irrigated with Neosporin eye drops. The inferotemporal area is most suitable for implanting the valve, but it can be placed in any quadrant.

CONJUNCTIVAL FLAP (5× TO 7× MAGNIFICATION)

A fornix-based conjunctival flap is created from 6 o'clock to 9 o'clock using a #75 Beaver blade (Fig. 11.3). Any scar tissue is excised, the conjunctiva undermined and the inferior rectus muscle isolated with a muscle hook. A 4-0 silk suture is passed

backward under the muscle hook and used to control the position of the globe.

INSERTING THE PLATE OF THE PROSTHESIS (5× MAGNIFICATION)

The conjunctiva is undermined posteriorly toward the equator, extending as far back into the fornix as possible. The plate is placed on the sclera under the conjunctiva (Fig. 11.4) and pushed toward the fornix until the anterior border lies at least 4 mm behind the limbus (Fig. 11.5). The positions of the anterior holes are marked with cautery on the sclera. Hemostasis of the entire area is obtained with wet field electrocautery.

A 9-0 nylon suture is placed through each anterior hole in the plate, and then an episcleral bite is taken where each cautery mark was made on the sclera. The sutures are tied, thus securing the plate to the sclera.

SCLERAL FLAP (5× TO 7× MAGNIFICATION)

A 3 mm square of sclera is outlined with a wet field electrocautery in front of the plate and extending from the limbus posteriorly in the inferotemporal quadrant. A one-half thickness scleral lamellar flap hinged on the cornea is dissected in this area using a #75 Beaver blade and a Grieshaber knife in the same way as for a trabeculectomy (Fig. 11.6). The dissection of the flap is carried to just inside the limbus (Fig. 11.7).

INSERTING THE TUBE OF THE PROSTHESIS (5× TO 7× MAGNIFICATION)

The anterior chamber is entered at the anterior border of the scleral flap through an entry incision made with a myringotomy blade or a #74 Beaver blade. The incision runs parallel to the plane of the iris. The tube is extended onto the cornea, measured and then cut so that approximately 3.5 mm of tube will extend into the anterior chamber. The tube is pushed into the anterior chamber through the limbal incision (Fig. 11.8) and protrudes for about 3.5 mm into the anterior chamber (Fig. 11.9). The tube is fixated by a 9-0 nylon suture placed through the scleral flap at the limbus through the tube and out

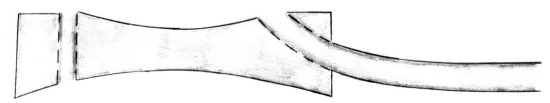
Figure 11.1. Seton. Side view of a Molteno implant shown diagrammatically. Note the biconcave shape, with the inferior surface shaped to fit the sclera. Anteriorly, the section cuts through the insertion of the silicone tube and posteriorly through the hole for a suture.

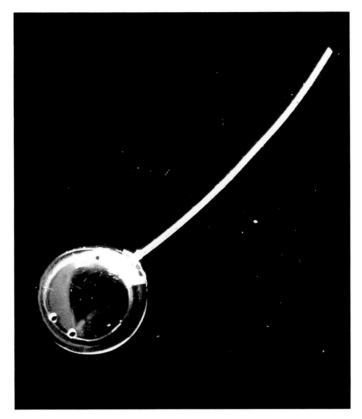

Figure 11.2. Seton. Photograph of a Molteno implant showing base plate and silicone tube.

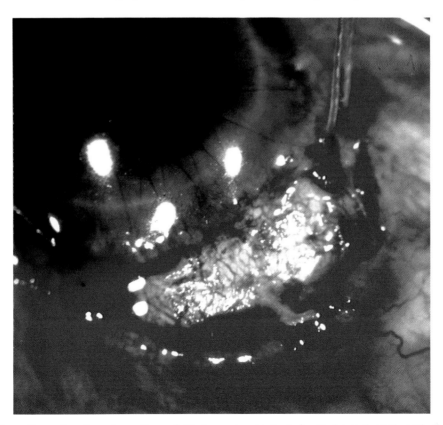

Figure 11.3. Insertion of seton. Insertion of Molteno implant. A fornix-based conjunctival flap extending over one quadrant is created.

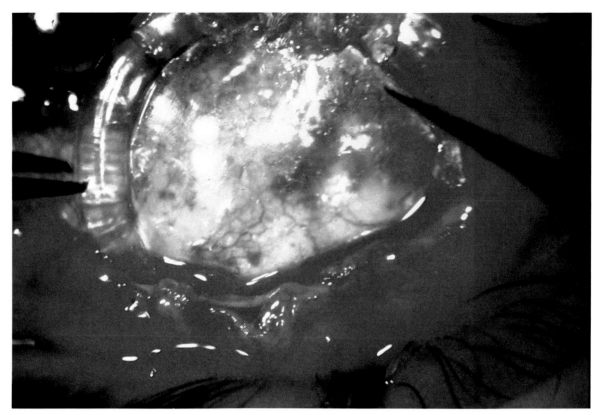

Figure 11.4. Insertion of seton (continued). The implant plate is placed on the sclera under the conjunctiva.

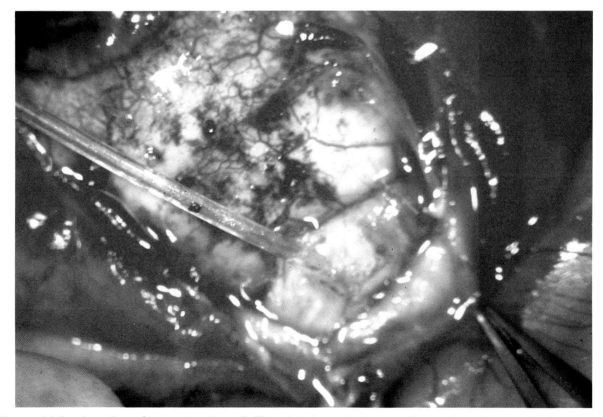

Figure 11.5. Insertion of seton (continued). The plate is pushed under the conjunctiva into the fornix until the anterior edge is at least 4 mm from the limbus.

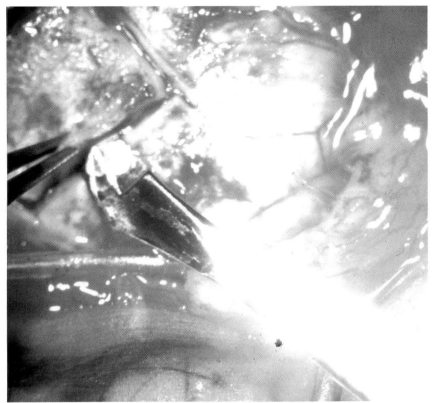

Figure 11.6. Insertion of seton (continued). A 3 mm square of sclera is outlined extending from the limbus posteriorly for 3 mm in the same quadrant as the implant.

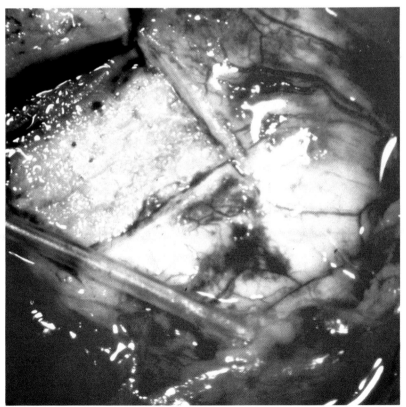

Figure 11.7. Insertion of seton (continued). The scleral flap is dissected from its posterior margin at one-half thickness depth to the limbus in the same way as for a trabeculectomy flap.

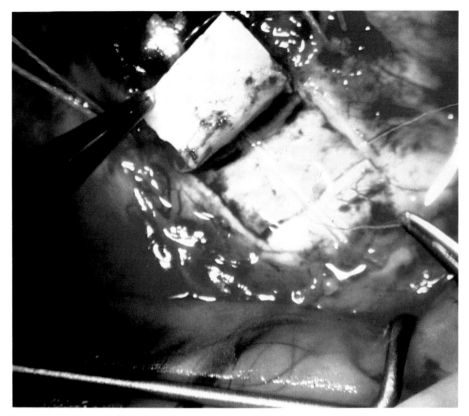

Figure 11.8. Insertion of seton (continued). The tube of the implant is pushed into the anterior chamber through this incision and fixated with 9-0 nylon sutures at the limbus and at the posterior edge of the scleral flap.

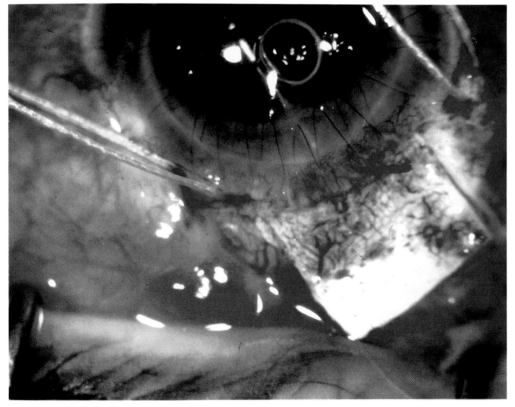

Figure 11.9. Insertion of seton (continued). The lamellar scleral flap is sutured back over the tube using interrupted 9-0 nylon sutures at the posterior corners and at the sides.

122

again through the scleral flap where it is tied. The lamellar scleral flap is closed at the sides with four interrupted 9-0 nylon sutures. The tube is then fixated to the sclera behind the scleral flap with one mattress 9-0 nylon interrupted suture, taking a bite of sclera on each side of the tubing. The tube should lie freely in the anterior chamber in front of the iris without touching the corneal endothelium.

CLOSURE (5× MAGNIFICATION)

The conjunctiva is closed with interrupted 6-0 plain sutures, one at 9 o'clock and one at 4 o'clock. Neodecadron drops are instilled in the eye. A pad and shield are taped over the eye.

Experience with the prosthesis extends over more than 5 years with good results. Molteno et al. (1979) use a two-stage technique rather than the one-stage technique described here, but the single-stage technique appears to give an equally good surgical result.

KRUPIN-DENVER VALVE

In 1980 Krupin et al. described the use of a seton with a pressure-dependent valve action. The technique, fully described in his report, is based on the use of alloplastic material fashioned as a seton and placed in the scleral fistula. The procedure has not been used long enough to evaluate adequately the long term results.

KREJCI-HARRISON SETON

This technique utilizes a strip of hydroxymethyl methacrylate (HEMA) which contains capillary tubules. The dehydrated sterile strip is inserted through a subconjunctival limbal incision into the anterior chamber, leaving a portion externally under the conjunctival flap. Rapid swelling on hydration fixates the seton. This seton has been used mainly in Europe with some success.

Chapter 12

COMPLICATIONS FOLLOWING FILTRATION SURGERY AND THEIR MANAGEMENT

Complications are seen in all filtering operations for glaucoma, but the incidence will vary according to the procedure and the status of the glaucomatous eye. The procedures with fewest complications are trabeculectomy, subscleral Scheie and subscleral trepano-trabeculectomy (see Chapter 8).

INFLAMMATORY REACTION IN THE ANTERIOR CHAMBER

Postoperative uveitis is the most common complication and in most cases is easily controlled with topical mydriatics and steroid drops. It rarely exceeds 2+ cells and flare and usually resolves by the end of the first or second week. Rarely, a severe postoperative uveitis becomes chronic and requires prolonged treatment. In such cases one should exclude other causes for the uveitis, particularly retinal detachment, trauma to the lens, an intraocular foreign body and systemic disease associated with uveitis, such as ankylosing spondylitis, chronic sinusitis or dental disease. Chronic uveitis must be actively treated to suppress the inflammation, and if this is not done the filtration area will be comprised by scarring.

FLAT ANTERIOR CHAMBER

A flat anterior chamber may be present on the first postoperative day but may be delayed until the second or third day. On slit lamp examination, there is contact between the iris surface and the posterior corneal surface. A chamber is usually present in the pupillary area because the anterior lens capsule and the posterior corneal surface are separated by interposed iris. The level of the intraocular pressure is all important. In flat anterior chamber due to excessive leakage from the drainage site, the intraocular pressure is low (less than 10 mm Hg). When the intraocular pressure is normal or higher than normal (21 mm Hg), it signifies a pupillary block glaucoma and/or "malignant glaucoma." Applanation tonometry in the presence of a totally flat anterior chamber will give false high readings which may lead to a mistaken diagnosis of malignant glaucoma.

Flat Anterior Chamber with Low Intraocular Pressure

There is a functioning conjunctival bleb due to excessive leakage of aqueous through the filtration fistula, or a "button-hole" in the conjunctiva of the bleb is recognized by a positive Seidel fluorescein test. Intraocular pressure is less than 8 to 10 mm Hg.

Prolonged flattening of the anterior chamber is a serious problem because the development of peripheral anterior synechiae leads to secondary glaucoma some weeks or months after correction of the flat chamber. Corneal endothelial degeneration and cataract are other possible complications.

The management is medically oriented for the first 5 days. If there has been no reformation of the anterior chamber after 5 days, surgical intervention is usually undertaken.

MEDICAL MANAGEMENT

Treatment is aimed at stabilizing inflow of aqueous and outflow through the fistula. This is attempted empirically by treating with a miotic (pilocarpine 4%) given 6 hourly, Diamox 250 mg twice a day and a firmly taped double thickness, oval eye pad. The miotic is discontinued after 24 hours if there is no response, and a mydriatic (Mydriacil 1%) is administered every 10 minutes for 2 hours and than q.i.d. The pupil often fails to dilate when the eye is hypotonous and the anterior chamber is flat. The rest of the treatment is not changed. After 24 hours, if there is still no response, the mydriatic therapy is abandoned and the patient is given 75 cc of glycerol 50% U.S.P. (Osmoglyn) b.i.d. flavored with fruit juice and over ice cubes. Steroid drops are continued. This regimen is usually successful. It may be repeatd for another 24 hours if the anterior chamber has not reformed provided there is no corneal stromal edema and there has been no actual lens-cornea contact. When these circumstances obtain at the onset, oral glycerol therapy is instituted without delay. Cataract will rapidly develop unless the anterior chamber is promptly reformed. Immediate surgical intervention is necessary if the central cornea remains in actual contact with the lens capsule for more than 24 hours.

Flat Chamber with Raised Intraocular Pressure: ("Malignant Glaucoma")

Malignant glaucoma is a rare complication of intraocular surgery usually seen after filtration surgery for angle closure glaucoma.

"Malignant glaucoma is defined as higher than normal intraocular pressure in an eye with a flat or shallow chamber and which usually follows surgery for angle closure glaucoma and does not respond to the routine surgery for glaucoma" (Duke-Elder, 1969).

The incidence is 2% to 4% of all operations for angle closure glaucoma. It may also arise after cataract extraction and during or after filtration surgery even when the angle is not very narrow or closed. The onset is likely to occur when steroids are withdrawn and if miotic therapy is instituted. The onset may be weeks or even months after the surgery. Malignant glaucoma can also develop prior to any surgical invasion of the eye, particularly in the presence of uveitis.

The anterior chamber is flat, the bleb may be well formed or flat, the pupil is semidilated and the iris is congested. Intraocular pressure is 15 mm Hg or more, rapidly reaching higher levels.

MEDICAL MANAGEMENT

Medical management is aimed at breaking the pupillary block by dilating the pupil and contracting the vitreous. Intensive dilatation of the pupil is undertaken by using a combination of mydriatics through a 12-hour period, for example Mydriacil 2% and phenylephrine 2.5% every 2 hours. These tighten the zonule and facilitate anterior chamber reformation. In addition, the patient should be given Diamox 250 mg b.i.d. to q.i.d. and 75 cc of Osmoglyn 5% (glycerine 50% U.S.P.) by mouth b.i.d. and, if necessary, intravenous mannitol 15%, 500 cc b.i.d. Topical corticosteroid drops will also reduce the inflammatory reaction and may assist in breaking the pupillary block or reducing ciliary body edema. Analgesics may be necessary. Topical therapy should be given only while the patient is awake, allowing adequate sleep during the night. If after 24 hours the situation is unchanged, surgical intervention is indicated.

Surgery for Flat Anterior Chamber (with Low or High Intraocular Pressure)

CONJUNCTIVAL "BUTTON-HOLE"

When the leak is at an area of conjunctival "button-hole," a small amount of Cyanoacrylate glue should be applied to this area, or with more chance of success, the leak is closed with one or two 8-0 virgin silk sutures. If this maneuver does not lead to reformation of the anterior chamber within 24 hours and there is still persistent leakage through the conjunctival hole, then the surgical procedure described below under "Rupture of Ischemic Bleb" should be followed.

FLAT ANTERIOR CHAMBER WITHOUT A CONJUNCTIVAL LEAK

Careful slit lamp examination of the conjunctiva and a Seidel test show there is no evidence of a break in the conjunctiva. One or more of the following mechanisms are the cause of the flat chamber and require correction.

Excessive Filtration through the Scleral Fistula

In trabeculectomy with a well sutured scleral flap, this is a very rare occurrence. The intraocular pressure is low, the iris surface flat and there is a large bleb.

Flat or Shallow Anterior Chamber with High Intraocular Pressure ("Malignant Glaucoma")

1. *Pupil block*, from a "tight" pupil or due to functional or organic adhesions between the pupil margin and anterior lens capsule (phakic eye) (Fig. 12.1) or vitreous face (aphakic eye) may result in the accumulation of aqueous in the posterior chamber; the iris becomes bowed (bombe) and is pushed onto the posterior corneal surface. It may drag the lens with it if it is attached to the pupil margin.

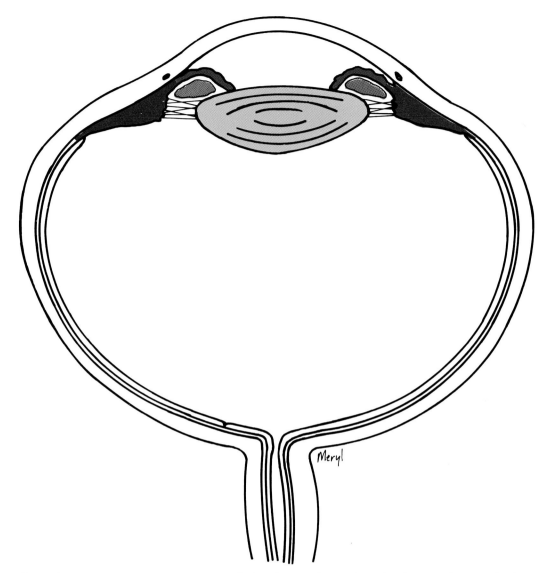

Figure 12.1. Pupil block "malignant glaucoma" showing pupil margin adhesions to the anterior lens capsule and the resulting increase of pressure behind the iris, causing iris bombe and angle closure. The result is a flat anterior chamber and high intraocular pressure.

Aqueous accumulates behind the iris, pushing the iris-lens diaphragm tighter against the posterior corneal surface (Fig. 12.1). Posterior vitreous detachment with compaction of the vitreous anteriorly and reduced permeability of the hyaloid to aqueous flow also facilitates the lens-iris shift forward. The angle closes, and the intraocular pressure rises. This condition is corrected by a laser or surgical iridotomy. In the event that the iridotomy or a scleral fistula becomes blocked by iris or lens, the intraocular pressure rises ("malignant glaucoma") and aqueous is pushed through the zonules and anterior hyaloid into the vitreous.

If the situation becomes chronic or develops slowly, the adhesions between pupil margin and anterior lens capsule (phakic eye) or anterior hyaloid (aphakic eye) may spread and result in extensive adherence of the posterior iris surface to the lens capsule (Fig. 12.2) or to the hyaloid face (Fig. 12.3). This gradual obliteration of the posterior chamber develops, and aqueous is forced back into the vitreous. In this situation fluid will be found only in vitreous and not behind the iris (Figs. 12.2 and 12.3).

This is recognized at surgery—peripheral iridectomy does not cause a free flow of aqueous from the posterior chamber. The posterior chamber must be re-established by separating iris from the vitreous face or lens surface if surgery is to be successful.

2. *Ciliary Block.* An engorged or anteriorly ro-

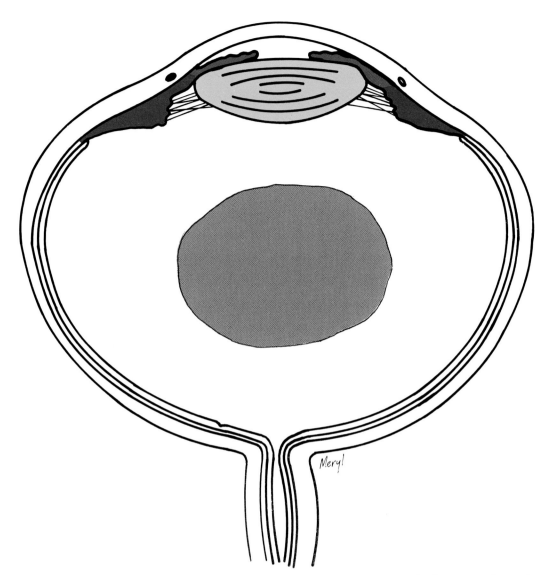

Figure 12.2. "Malignant" glaucoma. The iris has become adherent to the anterior lens capsule, and aqueous produced by the ciliary body is forced posteriorly into the vitreous. Fluid collects in the center of the vitreous, pushing the iris-lens diaphragm forward toward the cornea. The anterior chamber becomes shallow or flat, and the intraocular pressure is high. There is no iris bombe; the iris surface follows the contours of the anterior lens surface.

tated ciliary body may result in the ciliary processes moving centrally and clamping into the lens at the equator (Fig. 12.4) or onto an intact hyaloid. This obstructs the free flow of aqueous through the zonules, results in the accumulation of fluid in the vitreous and forms a vitreous pocket similar to the end result of a pupil block (Fig. 12.4).

3. *Suprachoroidal.* Another mechanism is by suprachoroidal fluid accumulation. Excessive filtration through the scleral fistula in the early postoperative phase causes exudation of the fluid from the choroid into the suprachoroidal space and results

in choroidal detachment (Fig. 12.5). These detachments will displace the lens-iris (phakic eye) or vitreous-iris (aphakic eye) diaphragm forward, and, if the detachments are large enough, the anterior chamber and posterior chamber are eliminated, forcing aqueous into a vitreous pocket. Unable to escape from the vitreous pocket, the accumulation of aqueous will push up the intraocular pressure in the presence of a flat anterior chamber.

A flat anterior chamber with high intraocular pressure is much more serious than a flat chamber where the intraocular pressure is low (less than 15

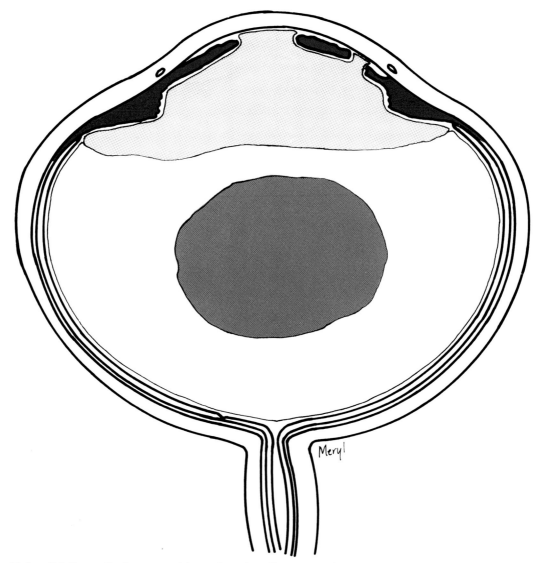

Figure 12.3. "Malignant" glaucoma. Iris surface is adherent to the anterior hyaloid face in an aphakic eye, aqueous collects in the vitreous, the anterior chamber is flat and the pressure is increased.

mm Hg) because corneal edema, endothelial cell decompensation and peripheral anterior synechiae ensue more rapidly.

The surgical correction of the flat anterior chamber is based on correcting these etiologic mechanisms. One or all of these mechanisms may be operative in any individual case.

"Malignant glaucoma" is unresponsive to glaucoma surgery. Surgical treatment is aimed at relieving the pupil or ciliary body block and draining fluid accumulation either in the posterior chamber (peripheral iridectomy) or vitreous. As it may be impossible to differentiate the causal mechanism, or more than one mechanism may be implicated,

the surgeon should be prepared to treat all possibilities.

Surgical Treatment of "Malignant Glaucoma"
LASER IRIDOTOMY

Where the anterior chamber is shallow but there is formed chamber over the total 360 degrees of the chamber, a laser iridotomy is performed (see Chapter 7). A successful iridotomy is instantly appreciated. The anterior chamber deepens, and the intraocular pressure drops. In the absence of a successful result with laser iridotomy, major surgery is necessary.

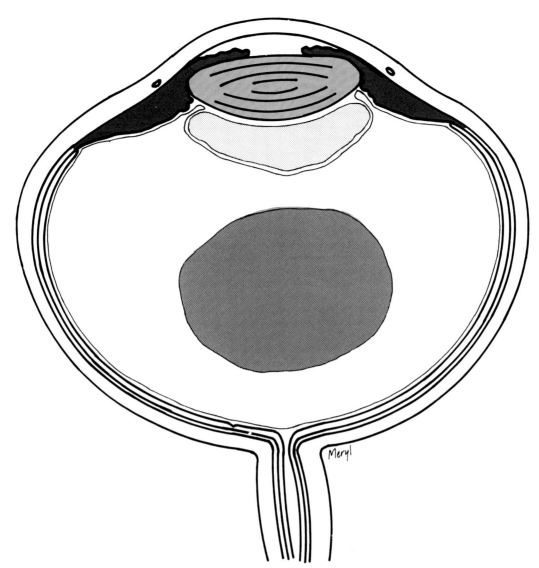

Figure 12.4. *a.* "Malignant" glaucoma. Diagram of engorged, anteriorly rotated ciliary body with ciliary processes clamped onto the lens equator. Aqueous produced by the ciliary body cannot flow into the posterior and anterior chambers. It is forced back into the vitreous, producing a pool of aqueous in the vitreous and resulting in "ciliary block malignant glaucoma."

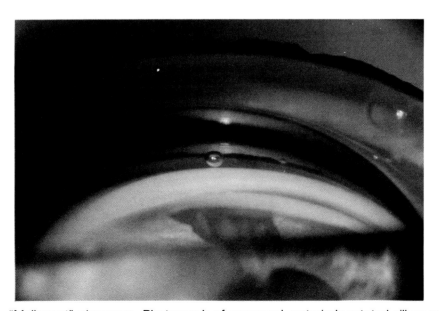

Figure 12.4. *b.* "Malignant" glaucoma. Photograph of engorged, anteriorly rotated ciliary processes seen through a peripheral iridectomy in an eye with "ciliary block malignant glaucoma."

129

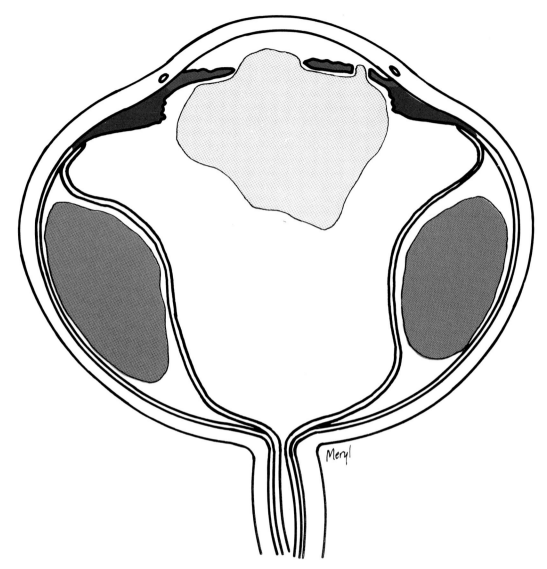

Figure 12.5. "Malignant" glaucoma. Accumulation of fluid in the suprachoroidal space, resulting in choroidal detachment. Fluid collection in this space may result from bleeding from the choroidal vessels (a mild "expulsive" hemorrhage or a choroidal effusion). Result is that the vitreous is forced anteriorly, the lens-iris diaphragm is pushed anteriorly and the intraocular pressure rises in the presence of a shallow or flat chamber, causing "malignant glaucoma."

PERIPHERAL IRIDECTOMY, POSTERIOR SCLEROTOMY, REMOVAL OF FLUID FROM THE VITREOUS

Preparation for Peripheral Iridectomy (7× to 10× Magnification)

Using a #75 microblade Beaver knife, a 3 mm long incision is made in the cornea just inside the limbus at the 6 o'clock meridian, and this is dissected to Descemet's membrane. The incision is preparatory to doing a peripheral iridectomy. The dissection is stopped at this point, and preparations for posterior sclerotomies are made.

Posterior Sclerotomy (5× to 7× Magnification)

A 3 mm long conjunctival incision is made parallel to the limbus and 3.5 mm behind the surgical limbus in both the lower nasal and lower temporal quadrants. At each sclerotomy site, the conjunctival incision is carried through the subconjunctival tissue to the sclera, cleaning all tissue off the scleral surface (Fig. 12.6). A cautery mark is made 3.5 mm behind the surgical limbus. Using a #75 Beaver knife blade, a 2-mm incision is made parallel to the limbus, incising through sclera at the surface of the pars plana (Fig. 12.7). Alternatively, 3-mm sclerot-

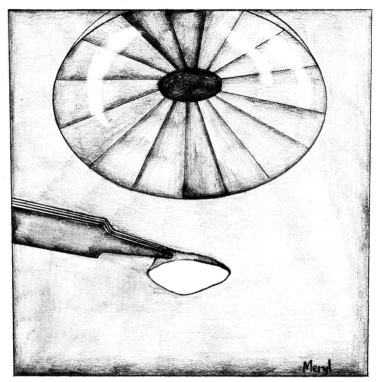

Figure 12.6. Posterior sclerotomy. A 3-mm conjunctival incision is made parallel to the limbus and 3.5 mm from the limbus.

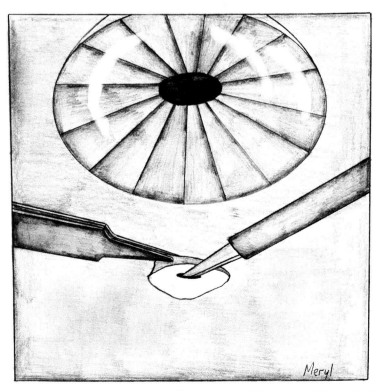

Figure 12.7. Posterior sclerotomy (continued). A 2 mm long incision parallel to the limbus is made in the sclera 3.5 mm behind the limbus. The incision is dissected down to the surface of the pars plana.

omy incisions may be made radially, centered at the 3.5-mm cautery marks.

Exploration of Suprachoroidal Space (7× to 10× Magnification)

As the surface of the pars plana is reached, search is made for a suprachoroidal fluid pocket. Unless there is immediate escape of suprachoroidal fluid, a flat spatula is carefully introduced into both sclerotomy incisions to separate pars plana from sclera and is pushed under the sclera for about 0.5 mm because suprachoroidal fluid occasionally loculates (Fig. 12.8). If no fluid is found, the sclerotomy in the lower nasal quadrant is sutured using one 7-0 Mersilene mattress suture with the knot tied away from the limbus. A mattress suture is placed in the sclerotomy incision in the inferior temporal quadrant using 7-0 Mersilene, and one knot is thrown but is only loosely tied. The suture material within the incision is withdrawn and placed aside from the wound (Fig. 12.10).

Paracentesis Incision (7× to 10× Magnification)

An incision in the cornea just in front of the limbus is made large enough to accept an air cannula (Fig. 12.9).

Iridectomy (7× to 10× Magnification)

The scleral side of the corneal incision at 6 o'clock is grasped with a #28 Hoskin forceps, and the cornea is pulled upward (toward the operating microscope). The assistant grasps the corneal side of the corneal incision and rotates this upward in the same way, thus exposing Descemet's membrane within the corneal incision and also stabilizing the cornea. Using the #75 Beaver blade, the surgeon completes the incision through Descemet's membrane into the anterior chamber. The iris may prolapse into the incision. If it does, a #28 Hoskin forceps (Keeler) is inserted through the incision, iris is grasped and a peripheral iridectomy is performed. The iridectomy must always be checked for patency. Fluid will drain through the iridectomy opening, the anterior chamber deepens and the intraocular pressure falls if there has been pupillary block.

When iris does not prolapse into the corneal incision but has to be pulled into the incision, then the surgeon should suspect that the posterior chamber has been obliterated by partial or complete iris-lens or iris-vitreous adhesions. This can be confirmed by completing the iridectomy and noting that little or no aqueous drains from behind the

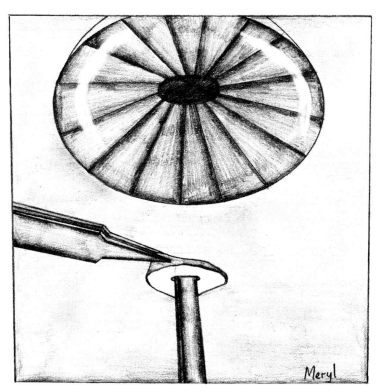

Figure 12.8. Posterior sclerotomy (continued). A flat spatula is introduced between the pars plana and the sclera into the sclerotomy site, and, with slight pressure on the pars plana, any fluid loculated in the suprachoroidal space will escape through the sclerotomy opening.

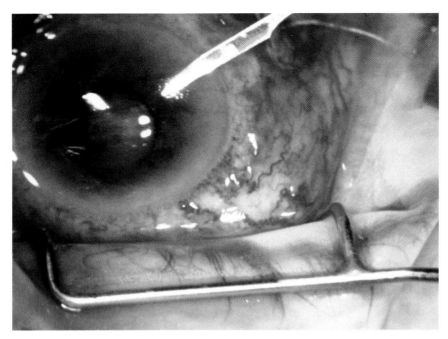

Figure 12.9. Posterior sclerotomy (continued). A paracentesis incision is made in the cornea just in front of the limbus, large enough to accept an air cannula. Photographed through the operating microscope at original magnification of 10×.

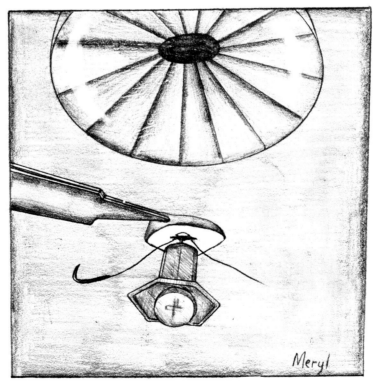

Figure 12.10. Posterior sclerotomy (continued). A mattress suture is placed in the sclerotomy incision to allow rapid closure. A 25-gauge cannula attached to a 2-cc syringe is introduced into the sclerotomy opening and through the pars plana, pointing it at the center of the globe.

iris. Lens capsule or hyaloid may be visible through the iridectomy, and the anterior chamber does not deepen. In this situation, an attempt can be made to free iris and pupil using a flat iris spatula, but it becomes mandatory to remove fluid from the vitreous through the previously prepared posterior sclerotomy.

The corneal incision is closed with one or two interrupted 10-0 nylon sutures, burying the knots on the corneal side.

Removal of Fluid from Vitreous (5× Magnification)

A 22- or 25-gauge straight cannula is attached to a 2-cc syringe. A point 12 mm from the tip of the cannula is marked off with a caliper, and a strip of Steri-drape is attached to the cannula at this point. The cannula is introduced into the vitreous cavity through the scleral incision, pointing the tip of the cannula toward the center of the globe and intro-

ducing it no further than (and preferably up to 2 mm before) the Steri-drape marker (Figs. 12.10 and Fig. 12.11). At the same time an air cannula attached to a Millipore filter and a 2-cc syringe filled with air are introduced into the anterior chamber through the previously made paracentesis opening. The plunger of the syringe is now withdrawn, and fluid vitreous should enter the syringe. At the same time, air is injected into the anterior chamber to avoid collapse of the globe (Fig. 12.12). If no fluid vitreous is found, the position of the cannula is changed slightly and another attempt is made to withdraw fluid. Approximately 1.5 to 3 cc of fluid vitreous are withdrawn, the cannula is removed and the scleral wound is closed by tightening the mattress suture and tying it. The conjunctiva is closed by interrupted 6-0 plain catgut sutures.

At this point, the eye is soft, and the anterior chamber is filled with air. The air is slowly removed

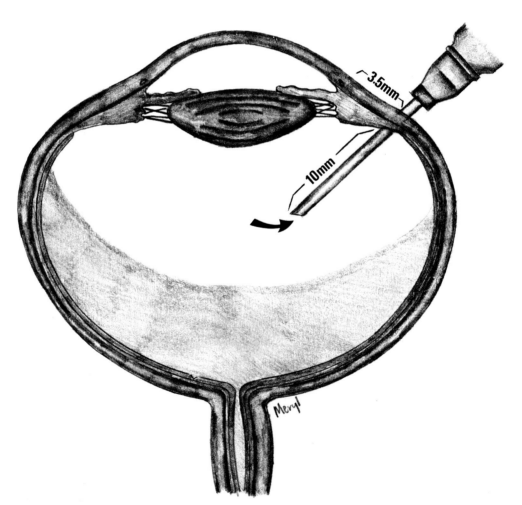

Figure 12.11. Posterior sclerotomy (continued). The cannula should be 12 mm long or has a Steri-strip marker attached 12 mm from the tip. The cannula is inserted no further than 10 mm into the vitreous body.

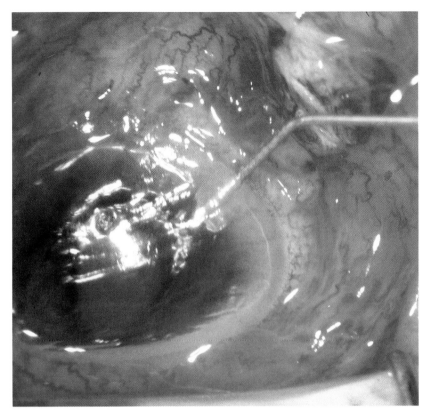

Figure 12.12. Posterior sclerotomy (continued). Air is injected into the anterior chamber through the paracentesis opening as fluid is removed from the fluid pocket in the vitreous through the 25-gauge cannula. This prevents collapse of the globe and maintains a reasonable pressure within the globe. Up to 2.5 to 3.0 cc of fluid can be safely removed in this way.

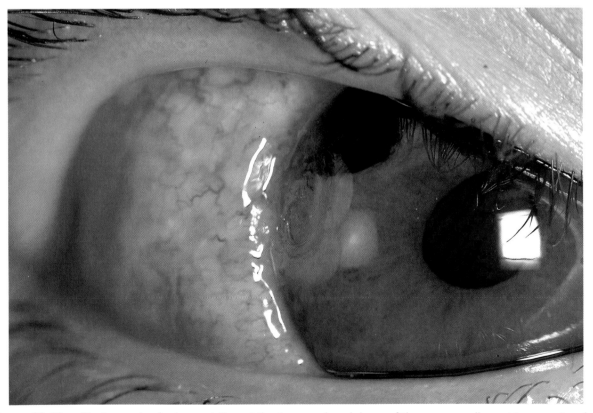

Figure 12.13. Photograph of a large dellen at the temporal periphery of the cornea adjacent to an extensive bleb from a trabeculectomy operation. The trabeculectomy was done on the temporal side because the patient had had previous filtration surgery on the superior quadrant of this eye. The size of the bleb prevents adequate lid massage of the cornea, leading to the dellen formation.

and replaced with just enough balanced salt solution to maintain the anterior chamber and a reasonable intraocular pressure (not above 10 mm Hg). The paracentesis does not require closure unless it leaks.

Postoperatively, a steroid-antibiotic combination eye drop is used for 3 to 5 days, depending on the postoperative uveitis. A short acting mydriatic to keep the pupil moving should be used only if there is significant uveitis.

Relapse

If the chamber again flattens after surgery, the posterior sclerotomy is opened, vitreous fluid is tapped and the anterior chamber is reconstituted with balanced salt solution through the original paracentesis incision. The pupil is maximally dilated. This procedure can be repeated two or three times if necessary, although this is a rare requirement if the trabeculectomy scleral flap has been adequately sutured. Following a Scheie operation, if such a refractory situation develops, one end of the scleral fistula is sutured with an interrupted 10-0 nylon suture, thus reducing the size of the fistula (7× to 10× magnification).

SHALLOW ANTERIOR CHAMBER

A shallow anterior chamber may be seen on the first, second or third postoperative day. The anterior chamber is very shallow, but there is no actual iris-cornea contact. The same risk exists of permanent peripheral anterior synechiae and secondary glaucoma as with a flat chamber, but the prognosis is better since the development of peripheral synechiae is slower. A persistent shallow anterior chamber can be treated medically for about 14 days before requiring surgery. Surgical intervention, although seldom necessary, follows the same stepwise procedure as described for a flat anterior chamber.

HYPHEMA

The incidence of hyphema is about 5%, presenting on the first postoperative day. The hyphema rarely reaches more than one-fourth the volume of the anterior chamber and usually absorbs within a few days. There is no specific treatment required unless the hyphema increases in size and causes secondary glaucoma. If that occurs, the hyphema should be evacuated. An attempt is made to find the source of bleeding (usually from the ciliary body) and to cauterize it.

FAILURE OF THE BLEB

Bleb failure is the most common cause of inability to control intraocular pressure postoperatively. Fi-

brosis occurs from the episclera and Tenon's capsule. Fibrosis is inhibited by using a fornix-based flap for trabeculectomy (minimum dissection of episclera and Tenon's fascia), careful dissection and separate suturing of Tenon's fascia and conjunctiva in a limbus-based flap.

Iris incarceration into the fistula can be prevented by ensuring that the base of the iridectomy is larger than the width of the fistula. This is possible in trabeculectomy and posterior sclerectomy, but it is not possible in a Scheie operation.

Surgical Treatment (7× to 10× Magnification)

Fibrosis of the bleb requires surgery. A sharp knife, e.g., a Graefe knife, is passed under the conjunctiva from the side of the bleb, or from the limbus in a fornix-based flap, pushing the knife into the bleb area and dissecting the bleb off the sclera, thus attempting to re-establish drainage. When this does not immediately re-establish the bleb, the conjunctival flap should be redissected at the site of the bleb, starting from the original incision and dissecting all fibrous tissue from the bleb area. The conjunctival flap is then sutured.

CHRONIC POSTOPERATIVE HYPOTONY

When hypotony persists postoperatively in the presence of a good anterior chamber and a well functioning bleb, this implies too rapid aqueous flow through the fistula or a thin conjunctival bleb. It has serious implications, especially the development of cystoid macular edema. Active treatment is required. This complication has not been encountered in trabeculectomy where the scleral flap is tightly sutured. When there is no demonstrable leak through the conjunctiva, a thin-walled bleb may be treated with cryotherapy (6 to 10 applications at −60°C for 30 seconds with the 3-mm tip). This often thickens the bleb and alleviates the hypotony.

Surgical Repair of Fistula (7× to 10× Magnification)

The bleb should be opened by an incision of the fornix if it is a limbal-based flap and by an incision at the limbus if it is a fornix-based flap. The filtration site is exposed, and the fistula is reduced in size by using interrupted sutures. In a Scheie procedure, sutures should be placed at either end of the Scheie incision to reduce its size by approximately one-third. In a trabeculectomy where the scleral flap has not been adequately sutured, more sutures should be placed to secure the flap tightly. The conjunctival flap is then replaced.

Another approach is to apply caustic chemicals, such as caustic soda (sodium hydroxide), to the margins of the bleb. This method is destructive and unpredictable.

LATE CATARACT DEVELOPMENT AND ITS TREATMENT

Some patients develop cataract within several months to a year following trabeculectomy. This is most likely to occur in elderly patients who have incipient cataracts at the time of surgery. The cataract may require extraction, depending on the degree of visual impairment and the status of the fellow eye.

The cataract is removed by a standard technique of the surgeon's choice. A site for the cataract incision should be chosen away from the bleb. The bleb is usually situated superiorly, and the ideal site for the cataract incision is over the temporal and inferotemporal quadrants, extending to just reach the bleb but not involving the bleb. An alternative site is an inferior limbal incision, but this has the disadvantage of being less accessible than a temporal incision, making the surgery technically more difficult.

A superior corneal incision in front of the bleb is not recommended since it must be made too far down in the cornea in order to avoid disturbing the bleb by the incision itself or the sutures. It may be difficult to obtain an incision large enough for good exposure. This approach results in a visible scar in the cornea.

Whichever method is used, there remains a 35% to 50% chance of losing a functioning filtering bleb following the surgical intervention. This problem has contributed to the increasing popularity of a combined trabeculectomy and cataract operation (see Chapter 8) when medical therapy and laser trabecular surgery have failed.

VITREOUS LOSS

Vitreous loss at the time of trabeculectomy is very rare (0.5%). This is prone to occur when the glaucoma is secondary to ocular trauma and the lens is subluxated. Our practice is to minimize the loss by immediately closing the lamellar scleral flap and repairing it with multiple 10-0 nylon sutures.

DELLEN

This common complication at the peripheral cornea in juxtaposition to the elevated conjunctival flap is a source of ocular irritation which can be troublesome for up to 3 months (Fig. 12.13). Treatment consists of topical steroids and/or ocular lubricants, such as Liquifilm Forte or Tears Naturale. Tear replacement alone is the preferred treatment.

RETINAL DETACHMENT

One instance of retinal detachment in an eye with a previous history of nonrhegmatogenous exudative retinal detachment and one case of rhegmatogenous retinal detachment following loss of vitreous have been encountered in 400 trabeculectomies (R. Harrison).

SCLERAL STAPHYLOMA

Occasionally, when a trabeculectomy scleral flap is left unsutured or only its posterior corners are sutured, and also in full thickness filtering operations, uncontrolled postoperative intraocular pressure may lead to formation of a staphyloma. This occurs at the site of the trabeculectomy flap or at the fistula where the sclera is weakened, particularly in a buphthalmic eye and in severe secondary glaucoma. If the staphyloma remains stable and does not enlarge, it is not treated. When it does enlarge, it must be surgically repaired.

Surgical Repair of Staphyloma (7× to 10× Magnification)

In the case of a trabeculectomy, the scleral flap must be sutured to the sclera. The sclera, if very thin, may be perforated during the surgical manipulations. This can be avoided by a preliminary posterior sclerotomy followed by dissection of the conjunctival flap, exposure of the trabeculectomy scleral flap and suturing the latter flap back to the sclera. An attempt should be made to push exposed uveal tissue back under the sclera as the scleral flap is sutured into place. If this is not possible, the exposed uveal tissue should be destroyed by cautery and the scleral flap then repositioned. The uveal tissue should not be cut because this may cause excessive and uncontrollable intraocular bleeding.

In the case of a full thickness fistula operation, a band of donor sclera or Teflon is pulled across the staphyloma to strengthen the sclera and is secured by interrupted sutures to normal sclera on each side of the staphyloma (Figs. 12.14 and 12.15). Covering the fistula with donor sclera or Teflon is not compatible with maintaining good aqueous filtration, but a small opening can be made, if necessary, in the donor sclera or Teflon to communicate with the original fistula.

THIN ISCHEMIC BLEB

A thin-walled avascular bleb requires careful observation and optional treatment with a broad spectrum antibiotic once daily. Intensive treatment with an appropriate broad spectrum antibiotic is mandatory if conjunctivitis develops. Cryotherapy

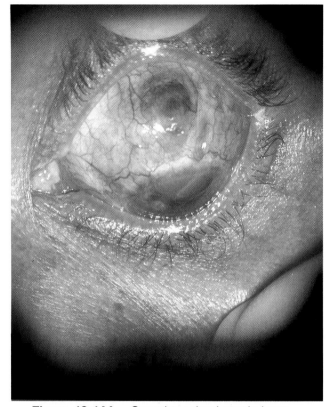

Figure 12.14A. Superior scleral staphyloma.

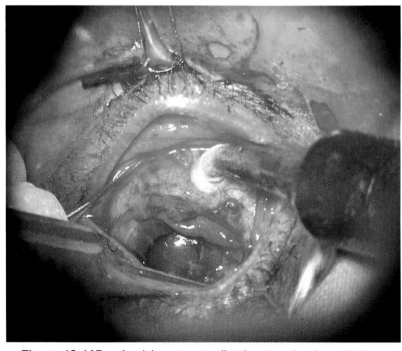

Figure 12.14B. Applying cryo application to scleral staphyloma.

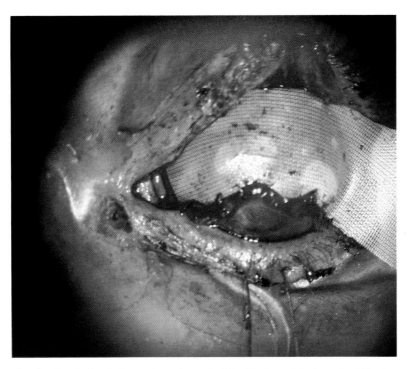

Figure 12.15. Repair of scleral staphyloma (continued). The Teflon strip is pulled firmly over the staphyloma and sutured to the opposite border of the staphyloma, covering the staphyloma and strengthening the sclera overlying the staphyloma.

to the bleb is indicated if there is a tendency to hypotony or leakage.

RUPTURE OF ISCHEMIC BLEB

Rupture of an ischemic bleb is a late complication of a limbus-based conjunctival flap. It is recognized by a shallow anterior chamber, low intraocular pressure and positive Seidel test at the site of the conjunctival fistula. Usually the patient notices a sudden drop in visual acuity. The eye is at high risk of developing intraocular infection. Surgical repair is mandatory if the fistula does not close within a few weeks, during which a topical antibiotic is used 4 times a day. Even when the fistula does close spontaneously, the conjunctiva will remain very thin, and a topical antibiotic should be used once daily indefinitely.

Surgical Repair (5× to 7× Magnification)

Local or general anesthesia may be used.

CONJUNCTIVAL INCISION

The conjunctiva is incised at the edge of the ischemic area to include and isolate the fistula. The line of incision is carried to the limbus and is extended for 3 to 4 mm on either side at the limbus, raising a fornix-based conjunctival flap.

CORNEAL INCISION

A one-half thickness corneal incision is made just anterior to the limbus, the length of the conjunctival flap. Cautery is applied along the base of the corneal incision, and a few applications are made on the anterior and posterior walls of the incision. The fornix-based conjunctival flap is rotated forward into this corneal incision and firmly sutured with interrupted 10-0 nylon sutures passing through, in series, conjunctiva, scleral lip of the incision, conjunctiva again, anterior lip of the incision and is then tied over the conjunctiva (Fig. 12.16).

Postoperatively, a topical antibiotic-steroid combination drop is used 4 times a day until the anterior chamber activity is minimal.

SEVERE POSTOPERATIVE UVEITIS

Inflammatory reaction of sclera, episclera and conjunctiva may be exceptionally severe and prolonged. Treatment is by topical cycloplegics and corticosteroids. Systemic steroids may be required, together with intensive use of topical steroids. Topical steroids are used until the inflammatory reaction subsides, which may take several months.

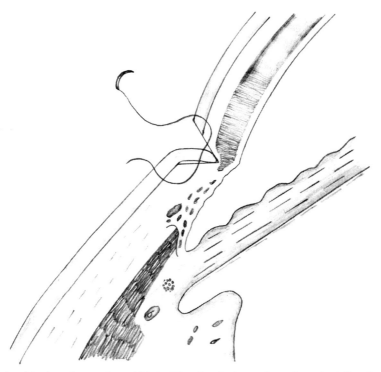

Figure 12.16.   Repair of ischemic, ruptured bleb. The fornix-based conjunctival flap is rotated forward into this corneal incision and firmly sutured with interrupted 10-0 nylon sutures passing through, in series, conjunctiva, scleral lip of the incision, conjunctiva again, corneal lip of the incision and is then tied over the conjunctiva. A similar procedure can be used with a limbus-based conjunctival flap after excision of the anterior portion including the fistula.

POSTOPERATIVE ENDOPHTHALMITIS

This is the most serious of the complications and has a poor prognosis for vision. The management involves aqueous and vitreous taps to establish the responsible organism. Systemic, subconjunctival, topical and, if necessary, intravitreal injections of antibiotics and corticosteroids are given.

This complication is often the sequela of a leaking ischemic bleb.

TENON'S-CONJUNCTIVAL CYST

Occasionally a prominent sausage-shaped cyst forms posterior to the limbus and the operative site, causing elevation of the upper eyelid and ocular discomfort. The intraocular pressure is often raised. Massage does not dissipate the cyst and does not lower the intraocular pressure. These cysts usually subside spontaneously after some months, and the intraocular pressure then falls to lower levels. Aspiration is rarely necessary (Figs. 12.17 and 12.18).

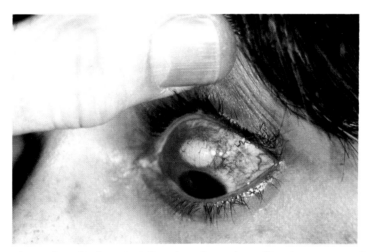

Figure 12.17. A Tenon's-conjunctival cyst at the site of previous filtration surgery. Note that inferior edge of the cyst does not reach the limbus.

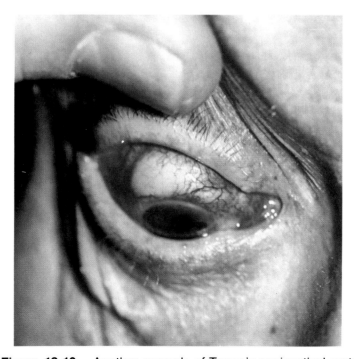

Figure 12.18. Another example of Tenon's-conjunctival cyst.

References

Abraham RK, Miller GL: Outpatient argon laser iridectomy for angle closure glaucoma: a two-year study. *Trans Am Acad Ophthalmol Otolaryngol* 79:529, 1975.

Alfano JE, Platt D: Steroid (ACTH) induced glaucoma simulating congenital glaucoma. *Am J Ophthalmol* 61:911–912, 1960.

Allen L, Burian HM, Braley AE: A new concept of the development of the anterior chamber angle. *Arch Ophthalmol* 53:783–798, 1955a.

Allen L, Burian HM, Braley AE: The anterior border ring of Schwalbe and the pectinate ligament. *Arch Ophthalmol* 53:799–806, 1955b.

Anderson B: *Hydrophthalmia or Congenital Glaucoma.* Cambridge, 1939.

Bain WES: *Br J Ophthalmol* 47:193, 1957.

Barkan O: Operation for congenital glaucoma. *Am J Ophthalmol* 25:552–568, 1942.

Barkan O: Goniotomy for the relief of congenital glaucoma. *Br J Ophthalmol* 32:701–728, 1948.

Barkan O: Surgery of congenital glaucoma. *Am J Ophthalmol* 37:1523–1534, 1953.

Barkan O: Pathogenesis of congenital glaucoma. *Am J Ophthalmol* 40:1–11, 1955.

Berger B: Dissertation, Tubingen, 1744.

Bigger JF, Becker B: Cataracts and primary open-angle glaucoma: the effect of uncomplicated cataract extraction on glaucoma control. *Trans Am Acad Ophthalmol Otolaryngol* 75:260, 1971.

Birge HL: *Trans Am Ophthalmol Soc* 50:241, 1952.

Boberg-Ans J: *Trans Ophthalmol Soc UK* 84:113, 1964.

Bonaiti C, Demonais F, Briard ML, et al: Consanguinity in multifactorial inheritance. *Hum Hered* 28:361–371, 1978.

Boyd B: *Highlights of Ophthalmology.* Panama, 1981, vol XVII, vol 11, 761.

Brochurst RJ: The IOP of premature infants. *Am J Ophthalmol* 39:808–811, 1955.

Burian HM, Braley AE, Allen L: Visibility of the ring of Schwalbe and the trabecular zone. *Arch Ophthalmol* 53:767, 1955.

Cairns JE: *Am J Ophthalmol*, 66:673, 1968.

Carvill B: *Trans Am Ophthalmol Soc* 30:71, 1932.

Chavand D, Clay CI, Pouliquen Y, et al: *Arch Ophtalmol* (Paris) 36:829, 1976.

Collins B: *Researches into the Anatomy and Pathology of the Eye.* London, 1896.

Collins B: *IX International Congress of Ophthalmology.* Utrecht, 1899, 88.

Coronet, Arnand: *Clin Ophthalmol* 18:498, 1912.

Curran EJ: A new operation for glaucoma involving a new principle of aetiology and treatment of chronic primary glaucoma. *Arch Ophthalmol* 49:131, 1920.

David R, Livingston DG, Luntz MH: *Br J Ophthalmol* 61:668, 1977.

D-Ermo F: *Albrecht von Graefe's Arch Klin Ophthalmol* 197:229, 1975.

deVincentiis V: Incisione dell angolo irideo nel glaucoma. *Ann Oftalmol* 22:540–541, 1893.

Douglas DH: Blindness in children of school group age. *Trans Ophthalmol Soc UK* 69:671–679, 1949.

Duke-Elder S: *System of Ophthalmology.* Henry Kimpton, London, 1969, vol XI.

Durr D, Schlegtendal F: *Albrecht von Graefe's Arch Ophthalmol* 35:88, 1889.

Eustace P, Harun AQS: *Trans Ophthalmol Soc UK* 94:1058, 1974.

Francois J: Aphatic glaucoma. *Ann Ophthalmol* 6:429, 1974.

Francois J: *Ophthalmologica* 177:158, 1978.

Frankelson EN, Shaffer RN: The management of coexisting cataract and glaucoma. *Can J Ophthalmol* 9:298, 1974.

Freedman J, Shin E, Abrahams M: *Br J Ophthalmol* 60:573, 1976.

Friedman AH, Luntz MH, Henley WL: *Diagnosis and Management of Uveitis: An Atlas Approach.* Baltimore, Williams & Wilkins, 1982, 107.

Galin M, Baras F, Perry R: Intraocular pressure following cataract extraction. *Arch Ophthalmol* 66:80–85, 1961.

Galin MA, Baras I, Cavero R, et al: Compression and suction ophthalmodynamometry. *Am J Ophthalmol* 67:388–392, 1969.

Gallenga B: *Ann Otolaryngol* 14:149, 1885.

Gregersen E, Kessing SV: Congenital glaucoma before and after the introduction of microsurgery. *Acta Ophthalmol* 55:422–430, 1977a.

Gregersen GI, Kessing T: The distended disc in early stages of congenital glaucoma. *Acta Ophthalmol* 55:431–435, 1977b.

Harrington DO: Cataract and glaucoma. Management of the coexistent conditions and a description of a new operation combining lens extraction with reverse cyclodialysis. *Am J Ophthalmol* 61:1134–1140, 1966.

Harrison R: Glaucoma in the aphakic eye. In Jakobiec F, Sigelman J: *Advanced Techniques in Ocular Surgery.* Philadelphia, W. B. Saunders, 1984.

Haut J: *Bull Soc Ophtalmol* 76:233, 1976.

Heath WE: Buphthalmos over three generations. *Br J Ophthalmol* 44:696–697, 1960.

Horner A: *Krankheiten d. Auges.* Tubingen, 1880.

Horven I: Tonometry in newborn infant. *Acta Ophthalmol* 39:911–918, 1961.

Hubner Z: *Augenheilk* 58:538, 1926.

Hughes WL: *Am J Ophthalmol* 48:1, 1959.

Hughes WL, Kasdan MS, Brackup AH, et al: *Am J Ophthalmol* 56:391, 1963.

Janesch G: *Albrecht von Graefe's Arch Ophthalmol* 118:21, 1927.

Jerndal T: Dominant goniodysgenesis with late congenital glaucoma. *Am J Ophthalmol* 74:28–32, 1972.

Jerndal T, Lundstrom M: Trabeculectomy combined with cataract extraction. *Am J Ophthalmol* 81:227–231, 1976.

Johns SC, Layden WE: *Am J Ophthalmol* 88:973, 1979.

Johnson JJ: Effects of routine extraction of the senile cataract upon the course of primary simple glaucoma. *South Med J* 61:865–868, 1968.

Kaminsky K: Hydrophthalmus congenitus. Thesis, Breslau, 1913.

Kaufman PL, Kolker AG: Ocular findings and corticosteroid responsiveness in parents of children with primary infantile glaucoma. *Invest Ophthalmol* 14:46–49, 1975.

Kayser N: *Klin Monatsbl Augenheilkd* 52:226, 1914.

Kestenbaum A: *Klin Monatsbl Augenheilkd* 62:734, 1919.

Khadadoust AA, Ziai M, Biggs SL: Optic disc in normal newborns. *Am J Ophthalmol* 66:502–504, 1968.

Kiehle FA, Pugmire C: Buphthalmos in identical twins. *Arch Ophthalmol* 12:751–752, 1934.

Kluyskens A: *Bull Soc Belge Ophtalmol* 94:4, 1950.

Komai BF: *Pedigrees of Hereditary Diseases.* Kyoto, 1934.

Krasnov MM: Microsurgery of glaucoma. Indications and choice of techniques. *Am J Ophthalmol* 67:857–864, 1969.

Krasnov MM: Laseropuncture of anterior chamber angle in glaucoma. *Am J Ophthalmol* 75:674–678, 1973.

Krejci L, Harrison R, Wichterle O: Hydroxyethyl methacrylate capillary strip. Animal trials with a new glaucoma drainage device. *Arch Ophthalmol* 84:76–82, 1970.

Krupin T, Kaufman P, Mandell A, et al: Filtering valve implant surgery for eyes with neovascular glaucoma. *Am J Ophthalmol* 89:338–343, 1980.

Laatikainen L: Late results of surgery on eyes with primary glaucoma and cataract. *Acta Ophthalmol* 49:281–292, 1971.

Lamb HD: Hydrophthalmus. *Am J Ophthalmol* 8:784–489, 1925.

Lehrfeld L, Reber J: Glaucoma at the Wills Eye Hospital, 1926–1935. *Arch Ophthalmol* 18:712–738, 1937.

Liaricos S, Chilaris G: *Ophthalmic Surg* 4:38, 1973.

Linn JG: Cataract extraction in the management of glaucoma. *Trans Am Acad Ophthalmol Otolaryngol* 75:273–280, 1971.

Lister L: The prognosis in congenital glaucoma. *Trans Ophthalmol Soc UK* 86:5–18, 1966.

Lohlein L: *Gutts Hb d Erbkrankheiten*, Leipzig 5:59, 1938.

Lowe RF: *Br J Ophthalmol* 51:727, 1967.

Luntz MH: In Turtz AI: *Ophthalmology.* 1969, vol 1, chap 9, 100.

Luntz MH: Congenital, infantile and juvenile glaucoma. *Trans Am Acad Ophthalmol Otolaryngol* 86:793–802, 1979a.

Luntz MH: *Doc Ophthalmol* 21:793, 1979b.

Luntz MH: Congenital, infantile, and juvenile glaucoma. *Ophthalmology (Rochester)* 86:793–802, 1979.

Luntz MH: In Boyd BF: *Highlights of Ophthalmology.* Panama, 1981, vol II, chap 37, 723.

Luntz MH, Berlin MS: *Trans Ophthalmol Soc UK* 533, 1980.

Luntz MH, Livingston DG: Trabeculectomy ab externo and trabeculotomy in congenital and adult onset glaucoma. *Am J Ophthalmol* 83:174–179, 1977.

Luntz MH, Schenker HI: *Surv Ophthalmol* 25:163, 1980.

Maumenee AE: The pathogenesis of congenital glaucoma.

Maumenee AE, Wilkinson CP: A combined operation for glaucoma and cataract. *Am J Ophthalmol* 69:360–367, 1970.

McPherson SD: Result of external trabeculotomy. *Am J Ophthalmol* 76:918–920, 1973.

McPherson SD, Dalton HT: Posterior form sympathetic opthalmia. *Trans Am Ophthalmol Soc* 73:251–263, 1976.

Merin S, Morin D: Heredity of congenital glaucoma. *Br J Ophthalmol* 56:414–417, 1972.

Molteno ACB: New implant for drainage in glaucoma. Animal trial. *Br J Ophthalmol* 53:161–168, 1969.

Molteno ACB, Van Biljon G, Ancker E: Two-stage insertion of glaucoma drainage implants. *Trans Ophthalmol Soc NZ* 31:17–26, 1979.

Molteno ACB, Luntz MH: *Br J Ophthalmol* 53:125, 1969.

Pare A: *Dix livres de chirurgie.* Paris, 1573.

Parsons JN: The refraction in buphthalmos. *Br J Ophthalmol* 4:211–216, 1920.

Paufique L, Sourdille PW: *Arch Ophtalmol* (Paris) 79:551, 1969.

Pfulger F: Ber Univ-Augenkli, Bern u d Jahr, 1882, Barrie, 1884.

Podos SM, Kels BD, Moss AP, et al: *Trans Am Ophthalmol Soc* 77:51, 1979.

Pollack IP: *Trans Am Ophthalmol Soc* 77:674, 1979.

Protonatarius P, Tsibidas P, Vassiliades J: *Isr J Med Sci* 8:8, 1972.

Raab A: *Klin Monatsbl Augenheilkd* 14:22,1876.

Randolph ME, Maumenee AE, Iliff CE: Cataract extraction in glaucomatous eyes. *Am J Ophthalmol* 71:328–330, 1971.

Rasmussen DH, Ellis PP: Congenital glaucoma in identical twins. *Arch Ophthalmol* 84:827–830, 1970.

Reis B: *Albrecht von Graefe's Arch Ophthalmol* 60: 1905.

Rich W: *Trans Ophthalmol Soc UK* 94:2, 1974.

Richardson KT, Ferguson WJ, Shaffer RN: Long term functional result in infantile glaucoma. *Trans Am Acad Ophthalmol Otolaryngol* 71:883–837, 1964.

Richardson KT, Shaffer RN: Optic nerve cupping in congenital glaucoma. *Am J Ophthalmol* 62:507–509, 1966.

Roberto W: Rapid progression of cupping in glaucoma. *Am J Ophthalmol* 66:520–522, 1968.

Robertson EN: Therapy of congenital glaucoma. *Arch Ophthalmol* 54:55–58, 1955.

Saint-Yves B: *Noveau traite des maladies des yes.* Paris, 1722.

Scheie HG: The management of infantile glaucoma. 62:35–45, 1959.

Scheie HG: Diagnosis, clinical course and treatment other than goniotomy. *Trans Am Acad Ophthalmol Otolaryngol* 59:309–321, 1955.

Scheiss-Gemeseus F: *Albrecht von Graefe's Arch Ophthalmol* 9:171, 1863.

Scheiss-Genuseus F: *Albrecht von Graefe's Arch Ophthalmol* 30:191, 1884.

Schwartz AL, Whitten ME, Bleiman B, et al: Argon laser trabecular surgery in uncontrolled phakic open angle glaucoma. *Ophthalmology (Rochester)* 88:203–212, 1981.

Seefelder M: Klinische und anatomische Untersuchungen zur Pathologic und Therapie des Hydrophthalmus congenitus. *Albrecht von Graefe's Arch Ophthalmol* 63:205, 481, 1950.

Seefelder M: *Klin Monatsbl Augenheilkd* 56:227, 1916.

Shaffer RN: Genetics and the congenital glaucomas. *Trans Am Acad Ophthalmol Otolaryngol* 69:253–268, 1965.

Shaffer RN, Hetherington S: The glaucomatous disc in infants. *Trans Am Acad Ophthalmol Otolaryngol* 73:929–935, 1969.

Shields MB, Simmons RJ: *Ophthalmic Surg* 7:62, 1976.

Smith P: *Trans Ophthalmol Soc UK* 16:348, 1896.

Smith R: A new technique for opening the canal of Schlemm. *Br J Ophthalmol* 44:370–373, 1960.

Smith RJ: Medical versus surgical therapy in glaucoma simplex. *Br J Ophthalmol* 56:277–283, 1972.

Spaeth GL, Rodriguez MM: *Ophthamic Surg.* 8:81, 1977.

Sugar HS: Symposium on secondary glaucoma: the congenital and infantile glaucoma. *Am J Ophthalmol* 33:1676–1680, 1950.

Sugar HS: Experimental trabeculectomy in glacuoma. *Am J Ophthal* 51:623–627, 1961.

Sugar HS: Experiences with some modifications of cyclodialysis for aphakic glaucoma. *Ann Ophthalmol* 9:1045–1052, 1977.

Sugar HS: The filtering operations—past, present, and future. *Int Ophthalmol Clin* 21:1–13, 1981.

Ticho U, Zauberman H: Argon laser application to the angle structures in the glaucomas. *Arch Ophthalmol* 94:61–64, 1976.

Villon JC: *Bull Soc Ophtalmol Fr* 76:693, 1976.

von Graefe A: *Albrecht von Graefe's Arch Ophthalmol* 15:108, 228, 1869.

von Graefe A: *Arch Ophthalmol* 3:456, 1876.

von Muralt U: Hydrophthalmus congenitus. Thesis, Zurich, 1869.

Walton DS: In Chandler, Grant: *Glaucoma.* Philadelphia, 1979.

Wechsler A, Robinson LP: *Aust J Ophthalmol* 8:151, 1980.

Wenaas EJ, Stertzbach CW: *Am J Ophthalmol* 39:71, 1955.

Wesbty RK, Skulberg A: Tonometry during general anesthesia. *Acta Ophthalmol* 40:186–191, 1962.

Westerlund E: On the heredity of congenital hydrophthalmos. *Acta Ophthalmol* 21:330–348, 1943.

Wilensky JT, Jampol LM: Laser therapy for open angle glaucoma. *Ophthalmology* (*Rochester*) 88:213–217, 1981.

Wise JB: Glaucoma treatment by trabecular tightening with the argon laser. *Int Ophthalmol Clin* 21:69–78, 1981.

Wise JB, Witter LS: *Arch Ophthalmol* 97:319, 1979.

Witmer R, Rohan JW: *Trans Ophthalmol Soc UK* 96:256, 1976.

Worthen DM, Wickham MG: Argon laser trabeculotomy. *Trans Am Acad Ophthalmol Otolaryngol* 78:371–375, 1974.

INDEX

Page numbers in *italics* denote figures; those followed by "t" or "f" denote tables or footnotes, respectively.